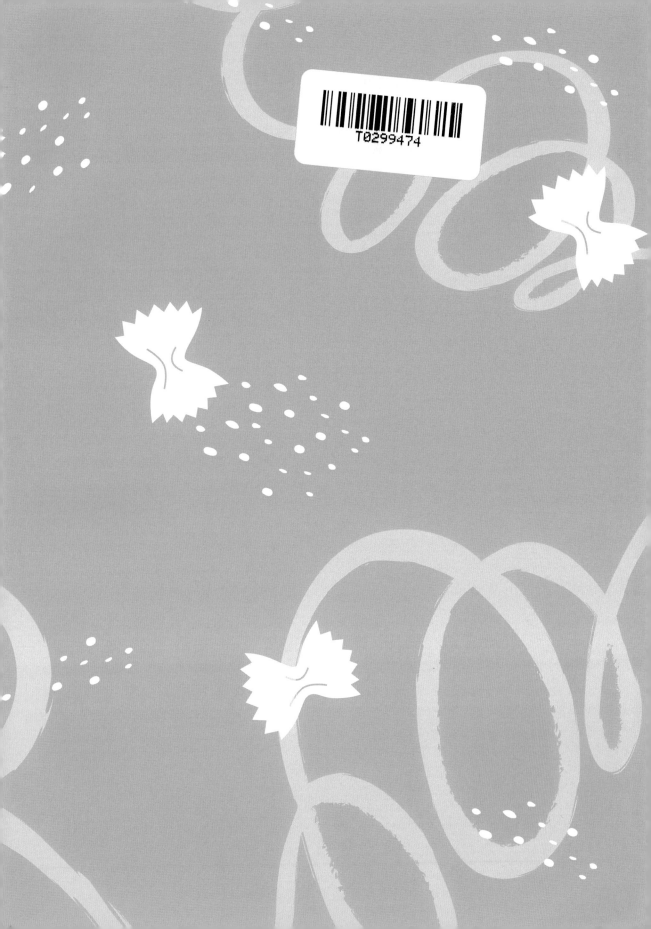

100 easy every day recipes for lunch and dinner

DELICIOUS GLUTEN FREE

Meals

SARAH HOWELLS

aka The Gluten Free Blogger

To everyone who's ever felt lost, alone
or disappointed eating a sad fruit salad
for dessert or a bunless burger for
dinner – this book is for you.

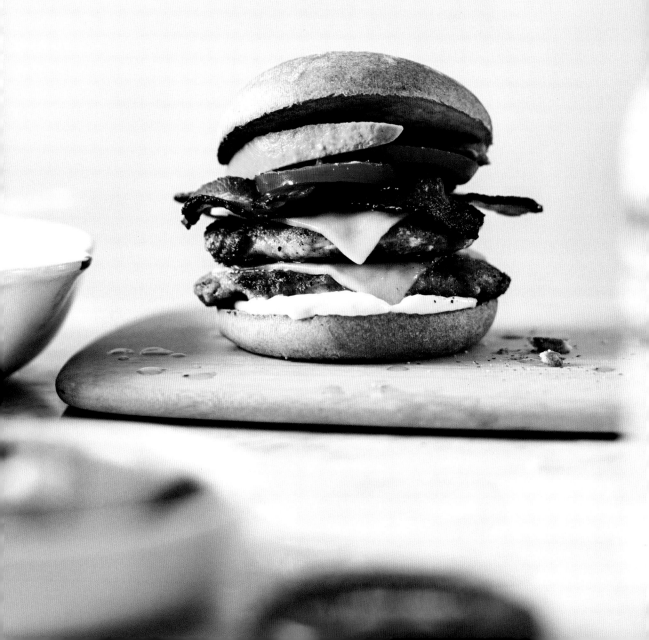

CONTENTS

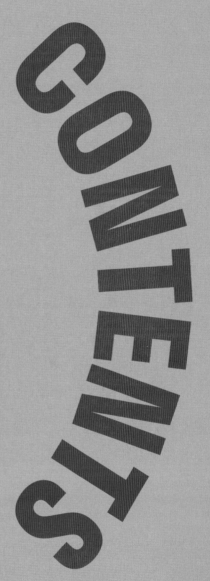

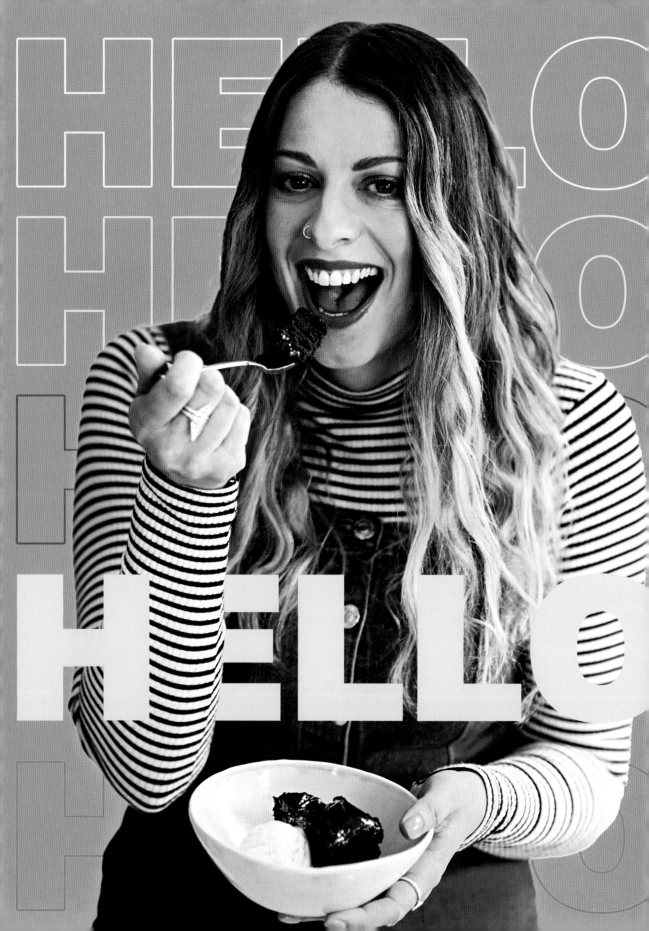

Introduction

Welcome to Delicious Gluten Free Meals, *the book that is about to transform your gluten-free life and save you from dry, tasteless, crumbly food forever...*

What's for dinner?

It's the age-old question that has fractured families, divided couples and broken even the hardiest of individuals. But when you're on a gluten-free diet, suddenly the question of what to cook for your next meal can become an all-consuming worry.

Well, not any more, thanks to this collection of delicious gluten-free recipes. I'm here to hold your hand through the process of becoming better at being gluten free, learning to love food again and, most importantly, never being stuck for ideas when it comes to deciding what to eat. Think of me as your gluten-free tour guide, and this book as your map.

New to gluten free?

Being told you have to go on a gluten-free diet can be a confusing and lonely experience. Often, after being given a diagnosis such as coeliac disease, you are sent out into the world and expected to just know what to do. As if giving up all the foods you previously relied on should just be easy.

And that's before you've filled your trolley with specialist free-from products and seen the cost.

Like all change, adjusting to a gluten-free diet takes time. You don't just ditch the bread for celery juice and #liveyourbestlife. Without the right help and support to guide you, it can feel like you suddenly have to give up not only all the foods you love, but the whole joy of eating.

Perhaps you're feeling lost on your quest to start a gluten-free diet?

Maybe you're standing in the bakery aisle, longingly staring at your favourite, freshly baked loaf and wondering how on earth you're going to keep up a gluten-free diet for life?

Do you want to be able to cook the same meal for everyone in your family without having to take out a second mortgage on your home or wash up a thousand different pans?

Or perhaps you're just so sick of only ever being offered a jacket potato as the gluten-free option that you're desperately browsing the bookshop in hopes of finding a solution?

'Oh, don't worry,' chirps the internet forum clique. 'Just cook everything from scratch, eat 15 portions of vegetables a day, meal plan for the next six months, only shop in the yellow sticker bin and eat naturally gluten-free foods forever and it'll be a breeze.'

But in reality? Life just isn't that simple.

Take it from someone who's spent many an after-work evening aimlessly wandering the supermarket on an empty stomach wondering what to eat that night. It's not just a case of grabbing a frozen ready meal or ordering a takeaway because, let's face it, that damn gluten gets everywhere. And what about the lack of grab-and-go lunch options, or easy breakfast ideas that aren't entirely based around the list of cereals you can't eat? As for the dessert menu, you might as well not even bother asking, unless you really love fruit salad.

Meals suddenly feel like they have to involve a lot of time, money and – dare I say it – effort. And it can feel a lot like you're missing out on all the foods you love. But let me stop you right there because that does not have to be the case at all.

The reality is, you just have to do things a little differently and you'll soon find you can still enjoy your favourite dinners, whether you have 20 minutes between tasks to throw together a plate of food, or a whole day to prepare a feast. Yes, you might have to learn a few new recipes and buy some ingredients you've never bought before, but let's think of it as a foodie adventure. Trust me, I've been where you are, and I want to help.

Not only is this book filled with all the recipes you need, it's also packed with information and tips to help your transition into a gluten-free diet – everything from learning how to shop and plan meals to save money, to talking to friends and family about cross-contamination.

This book is about to become the number one guest on your dinner party list.

I promise there is a way to happily eat gluten free and save money without having to be some sort of 5am-rising, caffeine-fuelled, Insta-worthy, meal-prepping 'hustler'. With the help of this book you're going to go from dreading every mealtime to looking forward to them. No more wandering the aisles looking lost and forlorn – it's time to get cooking!

Learning to cook from scratch can seem daunting, but not only is it going to help save you time and money, it will also make sticking to a gluten-free diet a lot easier. I might not be able to bring gluten back into your life, but I can help you bring back the flavour.

How to use this book

Starting with the fundamentals, we'll look at what gluten is (and what makes me so qualified to help you on this journey), how to tackle food shopping, making your kitchen a safe, gluten-free haven, and, of course, how to make 100 different gluten-free meals, sides and desserts that will rock your world.

I hope this book will become your well-worn kitchen assistant. I want you to scribble on it, add sticky notes, fold the pages and let it get splashed with food stains as you whip up your favourite recipe for the hundredth time. Hell, you can even write your shopping list in it and take it around the supermarket with you.

This is a book to be used and loved, and I hope it will provide you with a lifetime of happiness and full stomachs. Now, let's get cracking with the good stuff.

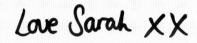

Love Sarah xx

My personal war against gluten

I know how much it can help to find someone who relates to what you're going through, so here's how I came to evict gluten – but not flavour – from my life, for good...

I had always been a skinny child, but the contradiction between my waif-like frame and my ability to demolish an entire box of cereal in one sitting and still be hungry soon became a concern. While my friends were starting to grow taller and curvier, I was a short and bony pre-teen with an almost constant gnawing stomach-ache. And despite always proclaiming my stomach pain had 'miraculously' disappeared every time I stepped into a doctor's surgery (much to my mum's embarrassment and frustration), we continued to investigate the problem.

There were a few attempts to alleviate my symptoms, including a short foray into eliminating lactose from my diet. But the stomach pains continued, and I still wasn't getting any taller. One day I saw a different doctor from my usual GP, who was off sick. This new doctor asked if I had been tested for coeliac disease, something that in those days was virtually unheard of. We had no idea what it was, but went ahead with a test anyway.

Coeliac disease essentially means the body attacks itself when you eat gluten, causing an antibody response that damages the lining of the small intestine. The disease has many different symptoms, which is probably why (according to the charity Coeliac UK) the average diagnosis time in the UK is 13 years. It's important to keep eating gluten to get an accurate result, so it was a good job I had still been eating my way through several boxes of cereal a week.

In 2002, at the age of 12, I was given a blood test that came back indicating coeliac disease-related antibodies. The next stage was to be referred for an endoscopy biopsy. I was given a general anaesthetic (though nowadays the test is usually done under sedation), and a sample was taken of my small intestine via a tube down my throat. A few weeks later, the biopsy results came back positive for coeliac disease and gluten was cancelled from my life forever.

Back then I didn't have the faintest idea what gluten even was. There were no shiny 'free from' signs beckoning me in the supermarket like an oasis in the desert. Instead, I was greeted with a solitary packet of coconut macaroons, which would later become my kryptonite after being the only gluten-free 'treat' served up at every party I went to for at least the next decade.

I often think of it as a blessing that I was diagnosed at such a young age. I hadn't yet learnt to cook and was still dependent on my parents, who took the full brunt of the learning curve like true champions. So while my mum spent hours scrutinising ingredient labels in the supermarket, I took the change in my stride, accepting that eating a different meal from the rest of my family was just the norm. Most of the time they graciously ate gluten-free meals at dinner time anyway, which made me feel much more included.

When it came to lunchboxes, I had never been keen on bread, cakes and biscuits, and I like to think it was my subconscious trying to steer me in the right direction. I didn't really enjoy many of the (limited) gluten-free lunch options back then either, and I'm pleased to say most things have come a long way since the days of cardboardy gluten-free bread.

It wasn't until I went to university that I think the full reality of being gluten free really hit me. There is no cure for coeliac disease. The only treatment is a lifelong, strictly gluten-free diet – the strict part being the bit I blissfully ignored during my first months away from home. But it only took a few rebellious, gluten-filled Chinese takeaways for me to realise that the pain they caused just wasn't worth it. Not to mention the potential, long-term complications that eating gluten could cause me if I carried on self-sabotaging in that way.

I started to realise it was up to me to look after myself now, and I quickly got used to cooking basic meals for myself, sticking to my diet without the support of my parents.

Thankfully, I'd picked up a few basic cooking skills while still at home and I put these to good use. But while I could now cope with the day-to-day management of being gluten free, it dawned on me that I had never actually met anyone else in my situation. And at times, that could be lonely.

Sometimes the burden of being gluten free was overwhelming, particularly when faced with a breadcrumb/gluten-coated student kitchen every single day. Or when everyone was going out for a meal somewhere that I couldn't eat at. My friends and family were always brilliant, but I felt like no one truly understood how I felt. I was studying for a journalism degree at the time, so when one of my lecturers suggested I start a blog to practise my writing, daily musings on my gluten-free meals seemed as good a subject to start with as any.

So in 2009, in my dingy student bedroom, *The Gluten Free Blogger* was born. Back then, Instagram didn't exist, blogs were only just starting to make a rumble online, and nobody had a clue that being an 'influencer' could be a career choice. I was merely sharing a food diary on the World Wide Web and hoping that others might relate.

But as I wrote, people responded. Suddenly a whole community of fellow gluten free-ers was reaching out through the tendrils of the internet, and for the first time I found people who could relate to how I felt. People who were just like me. What really struck me was how isolated a lot of these new online acquaintances also felt. And that was when I realised I wanted to establish and help a community of those starting on a gluten-free diet who had no idea where to turn.

The Gluten Free Blogger has come a long way since the days of me posting grainy photos of my questionable student meals along with ramblings such as, 'Dear diary, today I ate some pasta and it fell apart...' In fact, in 2019, a decade after my first blog

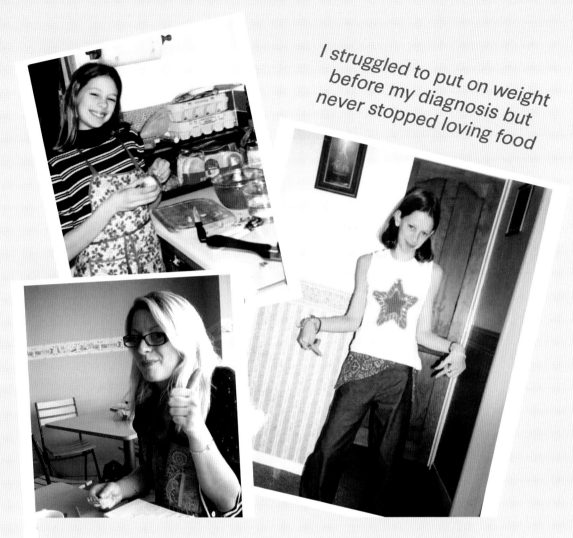

I struggled to put on weight before my diagnosis but never stopped loving food

post, I finally took the plunge to leave my job as a journalist and make blogging my full-time career.

However, the ethos of the blog, no matter how much it grew, has always remained the same, and always will – to help anyone struggling with a gluten-free diet and to build a community where nobody feels alone and no food is ever unattainable.

Not only did I find huge comfort in the supportive online community and make some amazing new friends, I also found happiness in learning to cook and bake for myself. I started to realise that cooking food from scratch was not only a lot easier than I ever imagined, but could be money-saving, made me more efficient with my time and

gave me an outlet to do something both physical and mindful. Cooking became my stress relief, eating became my joy, and sharing recipes with the gluten-free community became my purpose.

Nowadays the world is a much easier place to navigate for gluten-free people like us. Whole aisles bursting with free-from treats aplenty have opened up in supermarkets. There are entire restaurant menus (and even entire restaurants) dedicated to gluten-free food, and most people you know will nod with some sort of vague recognition when you mention the word 'coeliac'.

So trust me when I say: if I can do this, so can you.

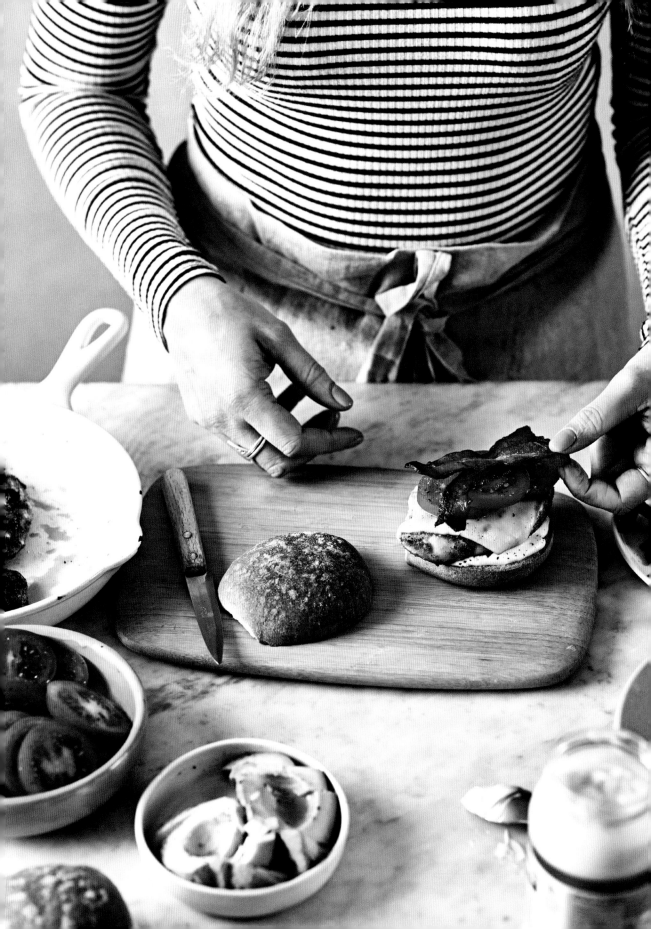

WTF is gluten?

Given we're here to talk about a gluten-free diet, it's probably a good idea to get a handle on what gluten actually is...

The chances are, when you first heard the word 'gluten', your mind went straight to a glue stick. And you wouldn't be completely wrong. Much as the name suggests, gluten – a protein found in certain grains – helps to form a glue-like consistency when mixed with water.

You know that lovely stretch you get when kneading dough? That's the gluten working its magic.

In fact, it's this very glue-like property that earned gluten its name in the first place. The protein is responsible for giving bread dough stretch and elasticity, helping it to rise during baking, and making the baked result so chewy and delicious. Those lovely big bubbles you see when you cut into a freshly baked focaccia? They're caused by the gluten allowing the dough to stretch as the yeast ferments. Basically, gluten is responsible for all the good stuff. But that's not to say it's irreplaceable. It just means we need to find a different way to make our favourite treats.

If you've already dabbled with gluten-free baking, you'll notice that it's not a case of simply switching out wheat flour for a safe alternative. Often this results in cakes that are dry and crumbly, biscuits that turn to dust in your hand, or pastry that sticks to everything when raw, then turns into a brittle mess when cooked.

Expecting a bread dough you can knead and shape? Think again.

Anyone who's tried to make gluten-free bread for the first time will remember the surprise (read: horror) of being faced not with a kneadable, stretchy dough, but a thick and gloopy batter. Remember, gluten really is the glue that holds so many bakes together.

So where exactly can you find gluten lurking? In short, it's found in the cereals wheat, barley and rye, and also in related grain products, such as couscous, spelt, semolina and bulgur.

What does this look like in terms of your shopping list? Turn the page to find a set of handy at-a-glance-guides to both the foods that contain gluten, and an abundance of foods that don't.

Common foods containing gluten

- Biscuits
- Bread
- Breaded or battered foods
- Cakes
- Cereals
- Egg noodles
- Flour
- Gravy
- Pasta
- Pastry
- Pizza bases
- Ready meals
- Sauces
- Sausages and burgers

Common drinks containing gluten*

- Ales
- Barley-based fruit squash
- Beers
- Lagers
- Oat milk (unless labelled gluten free)
- Stouts

The best way to remember which alcoholic drinks contain gluten is to think of BALS – Beer, Ale, Lager and Stout. Gluten-free versions are available from craft beer shops and online, and can sometimes be found in the free-from aisle.

Welcome to the realisation that these items form the basis of most Western diets. But before you grab the gin (thank goodness that's gluten free!), it's not all bad. As we get further into this book, you'll see that the list of foods you can actually eat is a lot longer than the lists above.

Remember, not every single food we eat consists of grains, and lots of foods are naturally free from gluten. While many processed products may contain gluten, many raw ingredients do not. And it's these, combined with specialist free-from products, that will end up forming a large part of your diet.

Common gluten-free foods*

- Beans
- Butter
- Buckwheat
- Corn (including polenta)
- Cheese
- Eggs
- Fresh meat
- Fresh fish
- Fruits
- Legumes (beans, peas, lentils)
- Millet
- Nuts
- Oils
- Potatoes
- Quinoa
- Rice
- Seeds
- Soya
- Sweet potatoes
- Teff (a type of millet)
- Vegetables
- Yoghurt

Common gluten-free drinks

- Cider
- Coconut milk
- Coffee
- Cordials
- Fruit juice
- Milk
- Nut milks
- Port
- Sherry
- Soya milk
- Spirits (gin, tequila, vodka, whisky)
- Tea
- Wine

While raw oats do not contain gluten, cross-contamination from other grains during the manufacturing process of both oats and oat milk can render them unsafe as GF products. Only oats labelled 'gluten free' are considered safe on a gluten-free diet, and the same rule applies to oat milk. Oats also contain a protein called avenin, which can cause a gluten-like reaction in people with coeliac disease, so, if you're eating gluten-free oats and still feeling unwell, it's best to speak to your doctor or dietitian.

Of course, as with everything in life, there are some caveats.

Buying fresh, non-processed foods from the lists above, such as meat, vegetables, rice and beans, is a sure way to guarantee you're eating completely gluten free. But many foods, as we know, have added ingredients or are processed in some way. And these are the foods that can blur the lines a little.

Naturally, you might find one brand of sausages is gluten free, whereas another is not. Or one supermarket may use gluten-free breadcrumbs on its fishcakes, while others don't. Of course, you should always double-check everything you buy to ensure it is gluten free (especially as manufacturers sometimes change the recipe of a food you've always relied on as being safe). The number one rule is never, ever assume, because we all know 'assume makes an ass out of you and me'.

Get ready to shop differently

Western diets revolve largely around gluten-containing foods, so it's natural to imagine you'll suddenly have to miss out.

Many of us were typically brought up to think a sandwich or wrap is the only appropriate lunch food. But what about soups, jacket potatoes, gluten-free wraps, salads, rice bowls or omelettes? Not to mention a trusty tub filled with delicious leftovers from your dinner the night before. These are just a few examples of some great lunch alternatives that can be had in place of a boring ol' cheese sarnie.

Once you learn which foods are gluten free and which are not, you'll find your world opens up in terms of food choices.

Supermarket sweep

Picture the scene: you've just been told to go gluten free, you're standing in the supermarket looking at the bread aisle where you usually pick up your staples and you're thinking *!*! (insert word I promised my mum I wouldn't write in my book). Where on earth do you even start when you're getting to grips with a gluten-free diet? At first it seems like everything contains wheat and the possibilities are getting ever narrower. But trust me, as you

learn how to navigate the food shop, you'll realise there are a lot more foods you *can* eat than foods you *can't*.

The best place to start is the free-from aisle, where all the gluten-free food hangs out. All the products here will be clearly labelled and anything with a 'gluten free' stamp will have been rigorously tested and audited to ensure it's genuinely free from all gluten.

But before you mine-sweep the shelves, delighting in the fact you can eat all these breads, cakes, pasta, biscuits and more, you might want to check the prices. Inevitably, all the extra precautions, less widely used ingredients and rigorous testing can come with a higher price tag.

When you're newly diagnosed, the free-from aisle is certainly an excellent place to start. It gives you an opportunity to discover what alternatives are out there, and makes you feel reassured that you won't have to suddenly give up all the foods you love. But while I recommend starting here and using it to get all your basics, the free-from aisle is not the be-all and end-all. Not if you want to avoid taking out a loan to fund eating.

Bulk-and batch-buying

Buying online from independent retailers can also be a great way to find new gluten-free goodies; for example, there are a number of mail-order bakeries offering fresh bread, cakes and more. But often they come with a minimum order, which is why I find buying these products in bulk and freezing them can work out more cost-effective.

The same goes with making your own gluten-free bread, meals and treats too. Most of these items can be frozen, so making a larger batch is often cheaper per portion, despite the higher initial outlay. This approach also helps to eliminate any food waste, which, let's face it, is just throwing money away.

Making friends with your freezer will definitely save you pennies and time. Batch-cooking things such as stews, sauces, pies and curries is a great way to ensure you have a go-to meal at hand without relying on overpriced gluten-free ready meals. Keep a stash of plastic tubs and labels so you can portion and mark up each meal with the name, amount and date of freezing. Unless, like me, you prefer to freestyle it, chuck a load of unmarked tubs in the freezer, forget what they all are and enjoy a bit of freezer roulette for dinner.

Learn to love food

For me, going gluten free meant learning to cook from scratch, and I regarded this as non-negotiable. While it was a steep learning curve, I find I now eat a much more varied diet. It's a chance to explore new products you never would have picked up before, and to try out new techniques and new ideas. Would you ever have looked twice at quinoa before going gluten free?

Would you have dabbled with baking your own bread if you could just buy it cheaply, or invested in a slow cooker if you simply relied on ready meals? Exploring food can be turned into a fun activity for all the family, challenging one another to find new ingredients you've never used before.

Cooking gluten free doesn't have to be restrictive or complicated; the joy is in finding ways to do it that suit your lifestyle and your wallet. I was as surprised as anyone to discover that I really do enjoy cooking simple and tasty meals.

Also, there's the added bonus that I can make things like pizza the size I want them to be, rather than settling for miniature gluten-free versions of the 'normal' food I used to eat. I might never answer the mystery of why all shop-bought gluten-free food portions are so tiny, but I certainly don't have to settle for them – and neither do you.

The bottom line?

I'll tell it to you straight: the first supermarket shop you do will probably be a struggle. And it's likely to be a bit of an eye-opener in terms of realising how much of the food you used to eat contains gluten. You'll make mistakes, you'll get frustrated when you see how many of your favourite foods are now a no-go, and you'll inevitably feel like this all sucks. But trust me, we've all been there, and that feeling soon fades.

As you start the habit of reading the ingredients of every single product in your cupboards and throwing half of them out (to a food bank, please), you'll also start to realise that you can do this. You'll start to understand what's gluten free and what's not. You'll begin to acquire new weekly favourites that you always buy, just as you did before you were gluten free, except now the shopping list might look a little different.

So what can you do to shop gluten free? Here are three tips to navigate the weekly food shop.

INGREDIENTS LISTS

The number one piece of advice I can give you is to learn how to read ingredient lists. That's because not every gluten-free product has to be labelled as such. Remember, manufacturers have to pay for testing to acquire GF status, so often products are safe to eat but not specifically labelled that way. You don't see 'gluten free' stickers on bananas or apples, but this doesn't mean they contain any gluten.

UK law states that common allergens in food products sold in shops must be highlighted in bold, so it's quick and easy to see if any gluten-containing ingredients are present. It's important to remember that the GF wording UK law specifies must be 'cereals containing gluten'. This means that while the word 'gluten' itself may not appear in bold, cereals such as wheat, barley, oats or rye could be highlighted instead. Unless the product is clearly certified as gluten free, the listing of any of these allergens means it's not safe to eat on a gluten-free diet.

'MAY CONTAIN' WARNINGS

While there are lots of naturally gluten-free ingredients available, if you have coeliac disease or a severe allergy or intolerance, you'll also need to be aware of 'may contain' warnings on food packaging.

These alert you to the fact that cross-contamination may have occurred during the manufacturing or packing of the product. In other words, the product you're looking at 'may contain' gluten.

For example, items such as polenta, spice mixes and quinoa are naturally free from gluten, but can have a warning stating they're made or packaged in a factory that also handles wheat. At present the laws around this sort of labelling are pretty open to interpretation, and therefore a source of great divide and frustration in the gluten-free community.

The general advice is to avoid products with 'may contain' warnings if you have coeliac disease. Unless, of course, you can establish directly from the manufacturer that the levels fall below the UK guidance of what is considered gluten free (20 parts of gluten per million). Otherwise. it's simply not worth the risk.

If no allergens are present but there's no GF seal of approval, double-check for 'may contain' warnings. If all clear, it's usually safe to go in the trolley. If you're still unsure, you can always check directly with the manufacturer. Scrutinising labels is the best way to come across goodies you never thought would be gluten free, or, as I like to call them,

accidentally gluten-free finds. You'll feel such empowerment when you seek out what's gluten free, rather than relying on the limitations of just one aisle for everything.

SHOP NATURALLY GLUTEN FREE

Now let's look at using products that are naturally free from gluten anyway. Think rice, potatoes, fresh meat and veg, and all the goodies from the long list on page 13.

Often, it will be cheaper to cook a dish with a side of rice than to find some certified gluten-free couscous alternative (which, let's face it, won't taste like you remember couscous to be anyway). And who doesn't love a potato, the most wonderful of naturally gluten-free carbs, whether it's mashed, roasted, fried or chipped? It is possible to do your entire shop without even visiting the free-from aisle – it just requires a little creativity. A number of the recipes in this book are naturally gluten free – **Aubergine Tagine** and **Chorizo & Cod Rice Pan**, for example – so you can use these as a starting point to put together meals without spending a fortune. I find this is also a better way to shop if you want to use local markets and farm shops, buying seasonal, locally grown produce and reducing the amount of processed foods (and air miles) in your diet.

Get those crumbs off my worktop!

You've mastered the art of food shopping, but how can you safely prepare your meals without accidentally getting glutened?

Perhaps the most overlooked aspect of being gluten free – particularly when you have coeliac disease – is avoiding cross-contamination. That is to say, the art of not mixing GF foods with gluten-containing foods and accidentally making yourself sick.

By this point you know how important it is to read product ingredient lists and 'may contain' warnings, so now it's time to consider how food can be safely prepared, cooked and served.

Preparing the kitchen

At first it might seem daunting to avoid cross-contamination while preparing gluten-free food yourself, but it's really just a case of common sense. In essence: don't let gluten touch any gluten-free foods. Simple, right?

Yes, if you're on your own, I hear you say. But what if you're catering for others? The easiest way to make sure you prepare a safe, gluten-free meal is to serve it to everyone else. A lot of the time non-GF people won't actually notice they're eating gluten-free food, so, when it comes to

meals such as Christmas dinner, it's pretty simple to stay safe.

If it's not possible to cook the same meal for everyone, there are a few steps you can take to limit cross-contamination:

- *Wash your hands and wipe down the worktops thoroughly before preparing any gluten-free food. Also ensure all the equipment you're using has been thoroughly cleaned.*

- *If possible, keep gluten-free food in its own cupboard or on a dedicated shelf.*

- *Where you have 'dusty' foods, such as wheat flour, which can easily spread, keep them in tubs or sealed bags in a different place from any gluten-free food.*

- *Always prepare gluten-free food on different chopping boards from gluten-containing foods, and use separate knives and utensils.*

- *Never put GF and non-GF foods in the same tray or pan. Use separate trays and pans, and always use separate spoons and spatulas for stirring and mixing.*

- If cooking several GF and non-GF items close together, watch out for any crumbs or splashes contaminating the gluten-free food. Things cooking on the *hob*, such as sauces and pasta water, can easily spit and splatter.

- Never cook gluten-free pasta or noodles in the same water as gluten-containing food. Always use fresh water, a separate colander and separate spoons to stir.

- If you're serving a buffet or help-yourself type of meal, ensure each dish has its own serving spoon and that the GF ones are kept separate. Double-dipping is a gluten-free person's worst nightmare, so it's a good idea to give them first dibs to avoid any accidents.

- Never toast gluten-free bread in the same toaster as 'normal' bread. Cheap toaster bags are a handy tool to avoid cross-contamination from crumbs without the need for a separate toaster (and they're useful for travelling too).

- In general, using the same pans, utensils, cutlery and crockery for GF and non-GF food is fine as long as they have been washed thoroughly. Utensils, such as sieves, can be tricky to clean, as can wooden spoons and tongs, which tend to absorb cooking ingredients. I always keep a separate set of these items for preparing gluten-free food. (Pro tip: paint the ends with red nail varnish so you can easily see which ones are safe to use.)

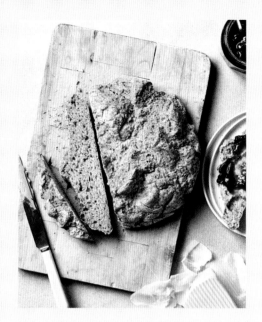

Shared kitchen spaces

Avoiding cross-contamination in a kitchen where only you cook is fine, but when you are living in shared or student accommodation it can be trickier. In my own university halls, I'm pretty sure environmental health officers would have had a hernia if they saw any food at all being prepared in the shared kitchens,

without even taking into account the potential for gluten cross-contamination. If possible, try to speak to your housemates and explain that you're not being fussy – you genuinely require a clean(ish) kitchen for your own health. It can be frustrating if you're always having to thoroughly clean up after everyone else just so you can make a sandwich, but sometimes it's a necessary evil when you're gluten free.

If your housemates aren't particularly understanding, there are a few things you can do that might help. In university halls I used to keep all my food and utensils in my room so I could lock them away and they wouldn't accidentally get contaminated if someone raided my cupboards in the kitchen. You could also consider investing in your own toaster, slow cooker, air fryer or small griddle to keep in your room. This will help to ensure it stays clean and gluten free.

Excessive as these precautions might seem, they could save you getting accidentally glutened and having to make a lot of extra bathroom trips. Also, once your housemates see the lengths you'll go to in order to keep your food and cooking utensils safe, they might start to take the situation a little more seriously.

Eating in non-GF houses

Mastered the art of cooking for yourself, but the idea of trusting someone else to do it completely freaks you out? It can be hard to hand responsibility to others, not just for reading ingredient lists properly, but for avoiding cross-contamination too.

Often, I find having a friendly conversation can be enough, explaining how important it is to keep everything strictly gluten free and not to take any risks. Once people understand it's for health reasons rather than fussiness, they will usually be eager to please and do what they can. When it comes to events or dinners, I always offer to bring a dish or dessert. This not only takes the pressure off the host to cook everything, but also ensures there is at least one thing I can eat that is gluten free. You can also volunteer to arrive early to help prepare the food, giving the host a helping hand and keeping a watchful eye over things.

If you can't get involved directly, invite your friend or family member to send you photos of products or ingredient lists if they need to double-check an item is gluten free. My friends often take me up on this, and they've all now become pretty savvy when it comes to knowing what I can and cannot eat. A few times they've even been shocked by what actually goes into some products, as they'd never bothered to read the ingredients before.

It's always important to approach the subject of your dietary needs in a calm way, as being demanding will instantly raise the hackles of whoever is cooking for you. And the last thing you want is someone angrily throwing food around the kitchen. Most of the time, your loved ones will want to make you feel included and will feel proud to be able to prepare a safe meal that you can enjoy. It can also help them understand exactly what you're dealing with and enable them to be more supportive of you and your dietary requirements. When

people are less accommodating, it can be hard to stand firm while not appearing difficult. I've found that if you stick to your principles, people will be less likely to take risks or make suggestions such as, 'Oh, just try a little bit.' Your health is the most important thing. If you have a difficult friend or relative who isn't being careful preparing your gluten-free food, simply decline the invitation. I know that feels harsh, but your health should always take priority.

Prepare your cupboards!

Before we get stuck into cooking lots of delicious food, here's a little overview of some of the common ingredients and equipment you'll need...

I know, I know – the recipes are so close that you can almost taste them, but before we start, it's time to sort out your cupboards. I believe it's really important that this cookbook provides affordable meal options, and that means stocking up on ingredients you can use time and again without any waste. Grab a load of these and you'll be able to turn to this recipe book whenever you're stuck for meal ideas without having to head out to the supermarket each time.

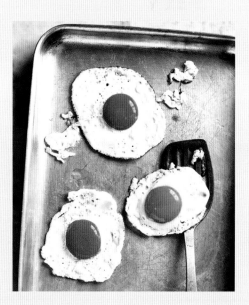

A letter to help you

Because I know how difficult dietary conversations can be, I've drafted a letter that you can show to friends and family who are catering for you. Feel free to rephrase it in your own words, or just give them a copy of this book, subtly adorned with sticky notes on all your favourite recipes. A friendly hint or two never hurt anyone, right?

Dear

First of all, I want to thank you so much for catering for me at
[insert awesome event/occasion here].

Having coeliac disease means the slightest cross-contamination can make me really unwell, and because of that, I know the idea of preparing a gluten-free meal may be a bit daunting. So here are some notes that I hope will make things a bit easier.

To avoid cross-contamination, any gluten-free food will need to be prepared and cooked separately from the other food, using separate pans and serving it in separate bowls (if we're having a buffet-style meal) with separate serving spoons. I am more than happy to help you with preparing the food if you'd like me to.

If there is any problem with avoiding cross-contamination, please do let me know. I'll happily bring a dish or two, as even a crumb in my gluten-free food could make me very unwell. I don't want to cause you too much difficulty, or ruin the fun by being ill or having to turn down your delicious food, so please let me help if I can.

I also know that understanding ingredient lists on food packaging can be a bit complicated sometimes, so please feel free to ask me any questions or send me a text or email with photos of products and their ingredient lists so I can double-check to see if they're gluten free.

A lot of supermarket products nowadays are gluten free as standard and clearly labelled, so hopefully the majority of the dishes you're making can be made gluten free anyway and nobody will even notice. I definitely recommend taking a trip to the free-from aisle in the supermarket, or having a flick through this book for some inspiration.

Thank you again for being such a wonderful friend/family member and catering for me. It means a lot to feel included.

Lots of love

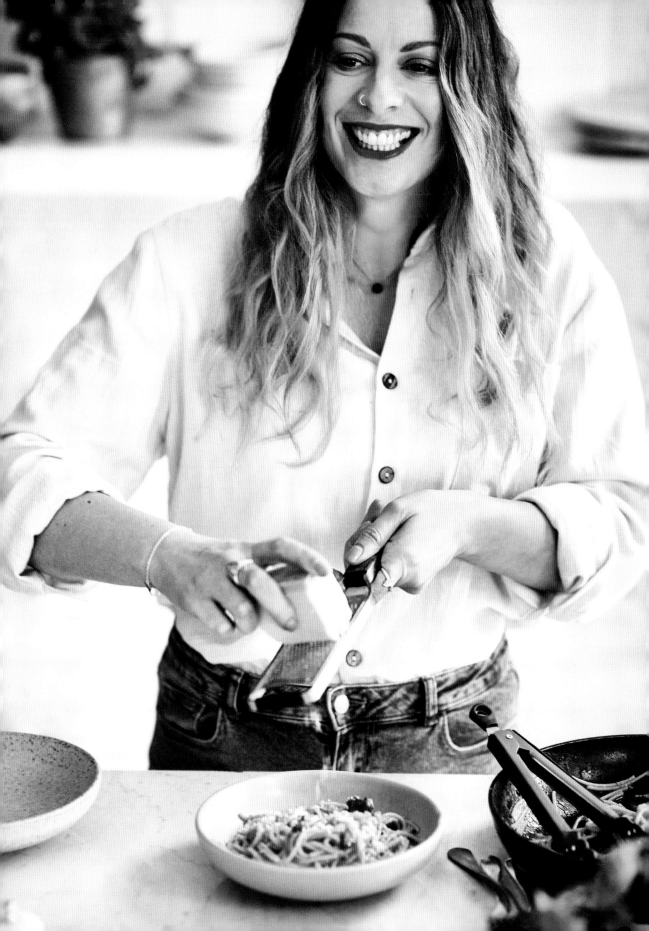

Here you'll find the common herbs, spices, store-cupboard ingredients and cooking equipment that underpin most of the recipes in this book.

Herbs and spices

There's nothing that winds me up more than finding you need to buy 16 different spices for one recipe, using half a teaspoon of each, and then never touching them again. To make life easier, nearly all the recipes in this book draw from the same collection of herbs and spices.

Listed below is the 'core stock' in my kitchen cupboards, which can be combined in various ways for all sorts of flavours. Once you've bought them for one recipe, you can use them for lots of others. As for the fresh herbs, you can either buy them in packets or pots from the supermarket, or even grow them from seed yourself. They make a lovely display on the windowsill and are close at hand whenever you need them.

DRIED HERBS & SPICES
- Basil
- Bay leaves
- Cayenne pepper
- Cinnamon (ground)
- Chilli flakes
- Chilli powder
- Chinese five-spice powder
- Cumin seeds (whole/ground)
- Curry powder
- Garam masala
- Garlic
- Italian mixed herbs
- Marjoram
- Mint
- Nigella seeds
- Onion salt
- Oregano
- Paprika (regular/smoked)
- Ras el hanout
- Rosemary
- Sage
- Tarragon
- Thyme
- Turmeric (ground)

FRESH HERBS
- Basil
- Bay leaves
- Chilli peppers (red/green)
- Coriander
- Mint
- Parsley
- Rosemary
- Sage
- Thyme

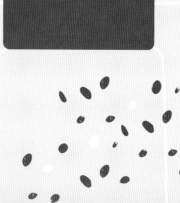

Store-cupboard essentials

As well as a good stock of the flavourings listed above, you'll also need a stash of other items to create lots of yummy, gluten-free meals and treats. You'll probably have many of these in your cupboards already, but do check they're genuinely gluten free.

BASICS
- Black pepper
- Gluten-free stock cubes and stock pots (beef/chicken/vegetable)
- Olive oil (regular/garlic-infused)
- Salt (table/flakes)
- Sesame oil (regular/toasted)
- Vegetable oil

BAKING NECESSITIES
- Baking powder
- Bicarbonate of soda
- Dried active yeast
- Gluten-free flours (chickpea/cornflour/ plain/self-raising/tapioca/white bread)
- Polenta
- Psyllium husks (whole)
- Sugar (caster/granulated/dark brown/ light brown)
- Vanilla extract
- Xanthan gum

PASTA AND RICE
- Basmati rice (dried/pre-cooked pouches)
- Gluten-free pasta shapes
- Gluten-free spaghetti
- Quinoa (pre-cooked pouches)
- Vermicelli rice noodles

BOTTLES, JARS AND TINS
- Chickpeas
- Chipotle paste
- Cocoa powder
- Coconut milk (full-fat)
- Garlic (chopped/paste)
- Ginger (ground/paste)
- Gluten-free Worcestershire sauce
- Harissa paste
- Honey (runny)
- Maple syrup
- Miso paste
- Mustard (Dijon/wholegrain)
- Peanut butter
- Red peppers (roasted)
- Sriracha
- Sweet chilli sauce
- Tamari (gluten-free soy sauce)
- Thai red curry paste
- Tomato ketchup
- Tomato passata
- Tomato purée
- Tomatoes (chopped)
- Vinegars (balsamic/red wine)

Equipment

Most of the recipes in this book require just a few basic items of kitchen equipment because I want everyone to find them accessible, no matter what you have in the way of hardware. Put simply, don't panic if you don't have exactly the right pan. Work with what you have and remember – necessity is the mother of invention, so you might find a better way to do something that works for you. In summary, here's the key kitchen equipment you'll need for most of my recipes...

- Baking paper (or reusable alternative)
- Baking trays
- Casserole dish (large, flameproof, with lid)
- Clingfilm (or reusable alternative)
- Colander
- Food processor
- Food thermometer
- Frying pan, large
- Grater
- Knives (good and sharp)
- Measuring spoons
- Mixing bowls
- Pie dish (23cm diameter)
- Roasting tray (large)
- Rolling pin
- Saucepans
- Scales
- Sieve
- Slow cooker (optional)
- Spatula
- Spoons (metal/wood)
- Stick blender
- Tongs

I'm very keen on a shortcut in the kitchen, and there are a few hacks I've learnt along the way.

DIJON MUSTARD: As English mustard is generally made with wheat flour, many people assume that other mustards are too, but that's not the case. Mustard flour, which is made from finely ground mustard seeds, contains no gluten, so Dijon mustard is nearly always safe, and a great condiment to add a flavour punch to your cooking.

GARLIC: Many of the recipes in this book call for chopped garlic, so I tend to prep and store a big bag of it in the freezer, which saves time on a day-to-day basis. If you want to do this, simply blitz some peeled garlic cloves in a food processor and freeze them to use as required. Of course, you can also buy jars of pre-chopped garlic and garlic paste. As a guide, 1 teaspoon of chopped garlic or garlic paste is equivalent to one garlic clove. Feel free to use whichever option is easiest for you.

GINGER PASTE: I always use jars of ginger paste. Chopped ginger is a good alternative and can be bought frozen or in jars. If using fresh root ginger, a 2.5cm piece – peeled, finely chopped or grated – is equivalent to 1 teaspoon ginger paste.

GLUTEN-FREE FLOUR: The two principal types are gluten-free plain flour and gluten-free white bread flour. If you cannot source the right product, they can be used interchangeably, but the result may be slightly different than intended.

SPECIALIST FLOURS: Some recipes, such as my gluten-free egg noodles, call for specific flours, such as tapioca flour. If you cannot source them from the supermarket, they can be ordered online from gluten-free producers. They will not go to waste, as they can be used for multiple recipes within this book.

LEMON AND LIME JUICE: I always opt for squeezing fresh lemons and limes, but using bottled lemon or lime juice will work fine if it's what you have. The bonus of leftover citrus fruits, though, is that you can slice them up and freeze them, ready for a G&T.

PSYLLIUM HUSKS: These are a form of plant-based fibre that becomes gloopy and gel-like when mixed with water. The mixture works really well in some gluten-free bakes where you need a little more flexibility in the dough. You can buy psyllium from health food shops or online – just make sure you get whole husks rather than the powder form, and double-check for 'may contain' warnings.

TAMARI: Chinese soy sauce is used in a lot of Asian cooking. but unfortunately for coeliacs, it contains wheat flour. Tamari is a Japanese alternative and nearly always gluten free, so I use it in place of soy sauce in my Chinese recipes and it works a treat.

XANTHAN GUM: Pronounced 'zan-than', this is an essential ingredient for gluten-free baking and can be found in most free-from aisles. It is a starch produced naturally by fermentation and often used in foods as a thickener. In gluten-free baking, xanthan gum helps to replicate the 'stretch' supplied by gluten. It is particularly crucial in bread and pastry recipes, as these often need to be rolled, stretched or proved. A little goes a long way, so a tub should last you for quite a while.

YEAST: In my bread recipes I used dried yeast rather than fresh yeast as it helps to speed up the process of making the dough. You can usually find it in the baking aisle of supermarkets, but always check that the product you buy is gluten free, as some brands are not. Fast-action yeast can also be used, but may need a shorter proving time than specified in the recipes, so follow the packet instructions.

Final pearls of wisdom

Before we get cooking, I'll leave you with a few pieces of kitchen wisdom I've learnt on my own through trial and error. I hope they'll help you to get the best from these recipes.

1 NO PEEKING!
If a recipe states to leave the lid on a pan, or to leave the oven door shut while something rests inside, try to resist taking a peek. Not doing so can release the heat or steam that's built up and slow the cooking time right down, which in turn can lead you to keep checking it even more and wondering why it isn't cooking. Trust me, it's a vicious cycle.

2 COOK ONCE, EAT TWICE:
I know I harp on a lot about batch cooking (I've even dedicated a whole chapter to it), but I can't emphasise enough how much time and money it can save. Buying ingredients in bulk is often cheaper and freezing leftovers means you won't spend out on pricey gluten-free ready meals, or struggle to find a takeaway you can eat.

3 TEST YOUR OVEN:
It's essential to preheat the oven before adding your food so it gets a head start. That said, it's unusual for an oven to be spot on in terms of temperature, so, if you feel your oven may be running hotter or cooler than it should, invest in a good oven thermometer to get the temperature right.

4 TAKE YOUR TIME:
Coming from the world's least patient person, I know this instruction is a bit rich, but I also know it's sensible. I've ruined more than one meal by whacking up the oven temperature when I was desperate to eat. Likewise, don't try to cram everything into one small pan if you have nothing bigger. It's far better to cook meat, for example, in batches so that it browns rather than stewing in its own juices.

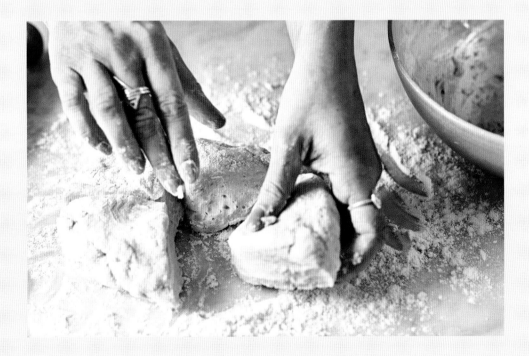

Let's get cooking!

You've swotted up on ingredient lists, cleaned the kitchen to within an inch of its life and stocked up the cupboards. Now, let's face it, comes the part we've all been waiting for...bring on the food!

I don't really believe in eating only certain foods for breakfast, lunch and dinner, so I haven't split this book up in that way, as many recipe books do. Instead, I cook according to how I feel. Do I need a quick and easy meal in under 30 minutes? Do I want a leisurely afternoon losing myself in constructing something slow and delicious, or do I want to avoid as much washing up as possible?

Here you'll find recipes to meet all those eventualities. We start, of course, with the basics – from a simple white sauce and GF breadcrumbs to pasta, pastry and tortilla wraps – which will allow you to create a variety of delicious gluten-free meals. After that, the recipes are divided into chapters to help you cook based on your available time and energy: everything from quick bites to slow-cooked dishes and wonderful desserts.

Of course, I had to include a few reader favourites from the blog, such as my **Cheeseburger Pasta**, the ULTIMATE pizza base and my **Cheesy Dough Balls**. But largely, I've filled these pages with brand new, delicious recipes that will replace all the foods you miss. I know being gluten free can feel like you're missing out, which

is why I've included GF versions of the meals you'd normally struggle to eat. From homemade gluten-free **Egg Noodles** to crispy **Fried Chicken**, golden **Steak & Mushroom Pie** and fresh **Cannelloni**, you'll never have to miss anything again.

The Quick and Easy chapter is the perfect place to dive in if you're short of time for everything from **Cheat's Chilaquiles** to **Fish Fingers**. If, on the other hand, you love the enjoyment of cooking, you can spend a leisurely afternoon in the Weekend Warmers chapter, cooking the likes of a gorgeous **Beef Stew** or **Chicken Casserole** with proper **Suet Dumplings**.

There's also a big focus on keeping gluten-free food affordable, whether you're batch-cooking a bolognese for the freezer, or enjoying some of the easy, naturally gluten-free options, such as my **Sausage & Sweet Potato Traybake**. Another big bonus is that from taste alone, you'd never guess that the recipes are gluten free. You can feed the whole family my **Classic Chicken Curry** or **Meatball Chilli Con Carne** or **Aubergine Tagine** and they'll be none the wiser.

Dietary information

At the beginning of each recipe are abbreviations that allow you to see at a glance what dietary needs, apart from GF, the recipes are suitable for. These are as follows:

DF **DF (Dairy Free):** These recipes don't contain any milk or dairy products.

DFO **DFO (Dairy-Free Option):** These recipes contain a simple ingredient switch to make them dairy free.

EF **EF (Egg Free):** No eggs are used in these recipes.

MF **MF (Meat Free):** These are perfect for vegetarians, and for those times when the rest of us might fancy a meat-free meal.

V **V (Vegan):** Free from any dairy, egg, meat, fish or animal products.

Number of servings

Almost all the recipes, bar a few desserts or meals that involve whole joints of meat, are designed to serve four people. However, if cooking for fewer than four, I recommend that you still make the full recipe and save any leftovers. These will provide a handy 'ready meal' that can be reheated or eaten cold. It's more cost-effective to do this than buying smaller quantities, and you won't find yourself having to think of ways to use up leftover ingredients.

Despite this advice, I know every household is different – some people may be cooking a feast for the masses, while others may be making a meal just for one – so that's why I've ensured it's easy to halve or double the quantities listed so you can cater accurately for the number of mouths you have to feed.

When I was growing up, my family made a huge effort to incorporate my GF needs into the meals that they were eating so I felt included rather than separate and peculiar. This approach is generally the cheapest and most efficient way of eating gluten free, far better than creating a separate GF meal for one person. It also made me very happy.

Cook's notes

While every single recipe in this book is completely gluten free, in some circumstances this depends on working with the right products. Where a listed ingredient could sometimes contain gluten (because brands differ in what they include), I've always specified a gluten-free version, such as 'gluten-free vegetable stock', not simply 'vegetable stock'. This is a reminder that you'll need to double-check such products before you buy them. Unless stated otherwise in the recipes:

- All spoon measures are level.

- All milk is full fat.

- All eggs are medium and preferably free-range.

- All vegetables (including garlic) are medium-sized and should be peeled or trimmed.

- All herbs and leaves should be washed and trimmed, as necessary.

- Sea salt flakes and freshly ground black pepper should be used wherever seasoning is required.

- I rely mostly on mild olive oil for cooking, and vegetable oils, such as sunflower and rapeseed, for deep-frying. That's because other types of oil can have a lower smoking point or create weird flavours. If shallow-frying, you can generally use any oil you like, including coconut oil, or even a 'light' spray oil. Reserve extra virgin olive oil just for salad dressings and drizzling.

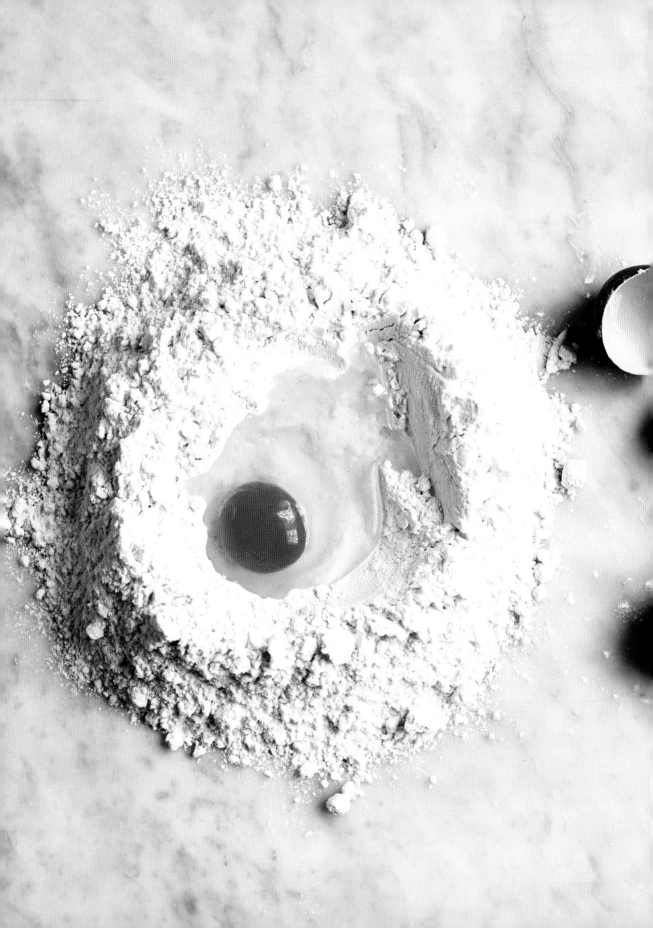

ABSOLUTE BASICS

Just as a good house must be built on strong foundations, it's important to base a gluten-free diet on sound basic ideas. Once you've mastered these basics, you can use them to create anything from simple snacks to a gluten-free banquet. This chapter guides you through these basic building blocks, which feature in many of the recipes that follow, so this is where the fun really starts. Think of it as a gluten-free crash course.

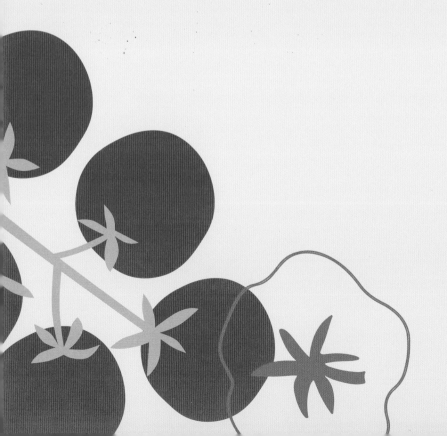

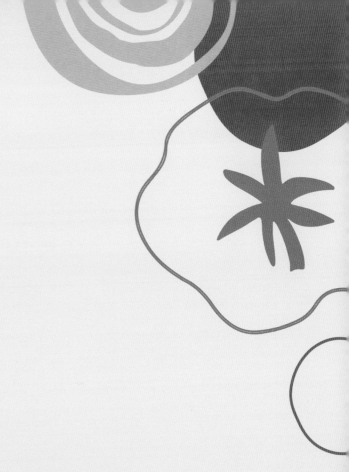

THE RECIPES

White Sauce

50g unsalted butter
50g gluten-free plain flour
500ml milk
Salt and pepper

Cook: **10 minutes**

A gluten-free white sauce, also known as béchamel, is something you'll need in your repertoire and use time and again. It forms the base of so many meals and can easily be flavoured with cheese, mustard, paprika, garlic or whatever you fancy. Be patient when stirring in the milk, and don't be tempted to slosh it all in straight away if you want a lump-free sauce.

Serves 4

1 Place the butter in a large saucepan over a low heat. Once melted, add the flour and whisk into a thick paste. Continue to cook for about 30–60 seconds, stirring constantly so it doesn't stick.

2 Pour in about 100ml of the milk and continue stirring until it forms a smooth, thick paste. Continue adding the milk about 100ml at a time, stirring constantly until smooth before adding the next lot of milk. You should end up with a smooth, thick white sauce.

3 Continue stirring until the sauce starts to bubble, simmer for 30 seconds, then turn off the heat. Generously season with salt and pepper and stir well.

This sauce works well with a variety of cheeses – try adding Stilton for a great broccoli cheese dish, Gruyère for a nutty flavour, or even a Mexican-style chilli cheese, depending on what you want to use the sauce with.

TOP TIP

As this sauce freezes really well, I sometimes make an extra big batch and freeze it in portions so I don't have to make it from scratch every time.

Easy Arrabbiata Sauce

2 tbsp virgin olive oil
30g butter or dairy-free alternative
4 garlic cloves, crushed
1 tbsp chilli flakes
1 tsp dried basil
2 x 400g tins chopped tomatoes (*see Tip below*)
1½ tbsp balsamic vinegar
1 handful fresh basil leaves, torn

Prep: **5 minutes**
Cook: **20 minutes**

If I can't decide what to have for dinner, or I'm feeling lazy, I'll almost certainly end up making this chilli-flavoured sauce. It truly is the hardest-working of all sauces, and can jazz up anything from meatballs and leftover chicken to your favourite vegetables or a tin of tuna. I always keep an extra portion in the freezer as a yummier alternative to a jar sauce.

Serves 4

1   Put the oil and butter into a large saucepan on a low heat and allow the butter to melt. Add the garlic, chilli flakes and dried basil and fry gently, stirring occasionally, for 2–3 minutes, until the garlic softens.

2   Add the tomatoes and balsamic vinegar to the pan. Stir and bring to the boil, then simmer on a low heat for 15 minutes.

3   Stir in the torn basil and your sauce is now ready to serve with gluten-free pasta for a perfect, simple meal.

TOP TIP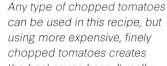

Any type of chopped tomatoes can be used in this recipe, but using more expensive, finely chopped tomatoes creates the best sauce base. It really is worth the extra investment. Failing that, you can also buy regular chopped tomatoes and finely chop them yourself before adding them to the recipe.

Gnocchi

1kg floury potatoes, such as
   Maris Piper or King Edwards
2 egg yolks

200g gluten-free plain flour,
   plus extra for dusting
Salt and pepper

Prep: **1½ hours**
(+ 30 minutes chilling)

Cook: **5 minutes**

DF

For something that is largely potato-based, gluten-free gnocchi is surprisingly hard to find in the supermarkets. Never mind – it's much cheaper to make your own, and rolling these little potato dumplings is oddly therapeutic. Some work off stress by going to the gym, others indulge in retail therapy, but I like to roll up little potato dumplings with a fork. Try it yourself and then tell me I'm wrong. Oh, and they taste amazing with an array of sauces too – which helps – a lot.

Serves 4

1 Preheat the oven to 180ºC/Fan 160ºC/Gas Mark 4. Place the unpeeled potatoes on a baking tray and bake for 1–1½ hours, until a dinner knife will go straight through.

2 Taking care not to burn your hands, transfer the potatoes to a board and cut them in half. Allow to cool slightly, then scoop the flesh into a pan, season with salt and pepper, and mash until perfectly smooth. This can be done in a food processor if you prefer. (You don't need the skins for this recipe, but they make a lovely snack if drizzled with olive oil and baked a second time until crisp.)

3 Leave the mashed potato to cool to room temperature. Once cooled, add the egg yolks and mix with a wooden spoon until combined. Sift in the flour and mix until a smooth dough forms.

4 Dust your work surface with some flour, turn out the dough and knead until smooth. Roll into a ball and divide into quarters.

5 Taking one quarter, use your hands to roll it into a long sausage shape about 2.5cm thick. Use a sharp knife to cut the sausage into 2.5cm pieces.

6 You can leave the gnocchi like this or, for a more traditional shape, take one piece at a time and gently press your thumb in the middle to make a dimple. After that, gently roll the dough over the back of a fork so that it slightly curls in on itself and has ridges across it.

7 When all your dough is shaped, lay the pieces out on a tray lined with baking paper, making sure they are not touching, and chill for at least 30 minutes.

8 Bring a pan of salted water to the boil and add the gnocchi pieces. Cover with a lid and bring back to the boil. As soon as the gnocchi float to the surface, about 2–3 minutes, remove them using a slotted spoon. Coat with the sauce of your choice and eat straight away.

TOP TIP

Get ahead by making and freezing a big batch of these gnocchi to use in recipes later in this book. The best way to do this is to freeze them spread out on a baking tray, then transfer them to containers or bags once frozen. I once accidentally froze a tub of gnocchi into one giant lump, so trust me, the flash-freezing method will save you an absolute headache.

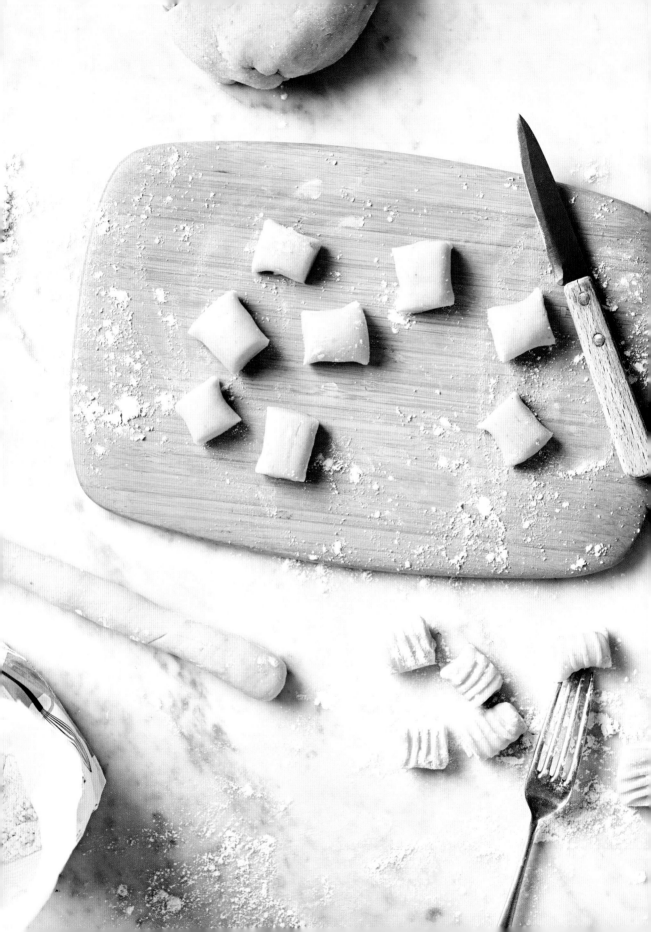

Fresh Pasta

200g gluten-free plain flour,
plus extra for dusting
2 tsp xanthan gum
2 large eggs, plus 2 egg yolks

Prep: **40 minutes**
(+ 30 minutes resting)

Cook: **8 minutes**

Sure, you can buy dried gluten-free pasta in the shops, but making your own is much more satisfying. You can also make it in a wider range of shapes than you can buy in the supermarket. I highly recommend using this recipe to make my Stuffed Cannelloni on page 108 – no one will ever know it's gluten free.

Serves 4

1 Mix the flour and xanthan gum together in a large bowl, then create a well in the middle.

2 In a separate bowl, lightly beat the eggs and egg yolks together. Pour them into the well in the flour.

3 Use a fork to mix the flour into the eggs until you have a ball of slightly sticky dough. Turn the dough onto a lightly floured work surface and knead for 1–2 minutes. It should form a smooth ball that is still a little tacky; if it's too sticky or wet, add more flour a tiny bit at a time.

4 Wrap the dough in clingfilm and leave to rest at room temperature for 15–20 minutes.

5 Divide the dough into 4 equal pieces. Wrap 3 pieces separately in clingfilm to prevent them drying out.

6 Generously dust your work surface with extra flour, then roll out the unwrapped piece of dough as thinly as possible, about 1–2mm thick. You can either cut it into rectangles to use as lasagne sheets or cannelloni, or use a pizza cutter or sharp knife to cut it into tagliatelle or linguine strips.

7 The pasta sheets can be used straight away for making lasagne. Tagliatelle or linguine can also be cooked immediately in a large pan of salted boiling water. Stir to ensure they don't clump together, and cook for 6–8 minutes, until al dente. Drain and serve with a favourite sauce, such as Easy Arrabbiata or Banging Bolognese (see pages 33 and 102).

Tortilla Wraps

250ml warm water
4 tbsp whole psyllium husks
300g gluten-free plain flour

1 tsp baking powder
1 tsp salt
30ml vegetable oil

Prep: **15 minutes**
Cook: **15 minutes**

 EF   DF   V

Who knew that making your own gluten-free tortilla wraps could be this easy? The secret lies in the psyllium husks – magical seeds that form a gloopy gel when mixed with water, helping to create a pliable dough. I love to make a big batch of these wraps and freeze them, ready to use in recipes such as my Mediterranean Quesadillas or with my Chicken Fajita Traybake (see pages 66 and 56).

Makes 8

1 Pour the warm water into a bowl, add the psyllium husks and mix well until a gel-like consistency begins to form. Leave for 1 minute.

2 Place the flour, baking powder and salt in a large bowl and stir together.

3 Pour the psyllium mixture into the flour, then add the oil. Use a wooden spoon to bring the mixture together and, when it becomes too stiff, use your hands to 'squish' it into a ball of kneadable dough. Keep going until there is no loose flour left in the bowl.

4 Divide the dough into 8 equal pieces, about 75g each, and roll them into balls. Set 7 of them aside and cover with a damp tea towel to make sure they don't dry out. Place the remaining ball in between 2 sheets of baking paper or clingfilm and roll into a circle about 20cm wide and 1mm thick, turning it regularly to keep it even. If you want, you can cut around a plate on the rolled dough to get a perfect circle, but I like to keep a 'rustic' look.

5 Place a dry frying pan on a medium-high heat. Once hot, peel the top layer of paper off the dough circle, then use the bottom paper to flip the circle into the pan. Peel off the paper and fry the wrap for 45 seconds on each side. It should puff up a little and develop some brown spots. If it starts to brown more than that, the pan is too hot, so lower the heat and set the pan aside to cool for 30 seconds.

6 Keep the wrap warm inside a tea towel, then cook the remaining pieces of dough in the same way. Keeping the cooked wraps together in a tea towel traps the steam and keeps them soft. Serve with your chosen fillings while still warm.

TOP TIP ▶▶▶▶

I recommend eating these wraps straight away. Although they can be stored for 2–3 days in an airtight container, you might need to refresh them with a 10–second zap in the microwave. You can also freeze them between sheets of baking paper to avoid them sticking to each other, then defrost and refresh in the microwave as needed.

Panko Breadcrumbs

Prep: **5 minutes**
Cook: **12 minutes**

EF   **DF**   **V**

Unlike fresh breadcrumbs, gluten-free panko breadcrumbs are crisp and dry, which means they absorb less oil when used to coat anything fried. It's virtually impossible to buy gluten-free panko breadcrumbs, yet they're unbelievably easy and quick to make – perfect for anything from pasta bake toppings to katsu curries.

Makes 150g

1   Preheat the oven to 160ºC/Fan 140ºC/Gas Mark 3. Line a large baking tray or 2 small ones with baking paper.

2   Cut the crusts off the bread and set them aside for now (see Tip below).

3   Blitz the bread slices in a food processor until they form crumbs. Pour them onto the prepared tray(s) and spread them into a thin, even layer.

4   Bake for 10–12 minutes, mixing them with a spoon halfway through. You're aiming for them all to dry out evenly, but not to brown at all.

5   Set aside to cool completely, then store in an airtight container, where they will keep for several weeks. You can also freeze them and defrost as needed.

TOP TIP

Don't waste the crusts – turn them into tasty, gluten-free croutons. Preheat the oven to its lowest setting. Cut the crusts into small cubes, then place in a bowl, drizzle with 2 tablespoons olive oil and season generously with salt and pepper. Toss to coat, then turn onto a baking tray in an even layer and bake for 10 minutes. For extra flavour, try adding garlic granules, onion salt or mixed herbs to the basic mixture. Use your gluten-free croutons in soup or salads.

Shortcrust Pastry

2 tsp xanthan gum
Pinch of salt
1 tbsp caster sugar (optional)
220g cold unsalted butter

3 eggs
2 tsp cold water
340g gluten-free plain flour,
    plus extra for dusting

Prep: **15 minutes**
(+ 30 minutes chilling)

Gluten-free pastry is the Holy Grail of GF baking skills, and a million times easier than you might think. I like to make this the old-fashioned way, using my hands, but this recipe works just as well in a food processor. It's perfect for all the gluten-free pies, pasties, tarts and quiches of your dreams. Halve the quantities if making a tart or quiche without a lid.

Makes 1 x 20cm pastry case and lid, or 2 cases without lids

1 Place the flour, xanthan gum and salt in a large bowl, adding the sugar only if making sweet pastry. Stir together.

2 Cut the cold butter into cubes and add to the bowl. Using your fingers, rub the butter into the flour mixture until it resembles breadcrumbs.

3 Crack 2 of the eggs into a bowl or mug and add the cold water. Whisk lightly until just combined. Pour into the flour bowl and mix with a fork until a sticky dough starts to form.

4 Once it becomes harder to use the fork, use your hands to bring the mixture together into a smooth dough, 'squishing' it well. You should be able to pick it up easily without it feeling too sticky.

5 Wrap the dough in clingfilm and chill for at least 30 minutes. This is really important, as it makes the dough easier to roll.

6 Once cold, use the dough as required.

BLIND BAKING A PASTRY CASE

- Line the case with a piece of crumpled baking paper and fill with baking beans, uncooked rice or dried lentils.

- Bake for 10 minutes in an oven preheated to 180ºC/Fan 160ºC/ Gas Mark 4, then carefully remove the baking paper and beans, and bake for another 5–10 minutes, until golden.

- Fill and bake the pastry case as per the recipe you're following.

TOP TIP

This gluten-free pastry can be wrapped and frozen for up to 3 months. Simply defrost and roll it out when you get a craving for a pie.

Rough Puff Pastry

250g gluten-free plain flour, plus extra for dusting
1½ tsp xanthan gum

250g cold unsalted butter, cut into 2cm cubes
1 tsp salt
150ml ice-cold water

Prep: **15 minutes (+ 1-1½ hours chilling)**

Perfect for sausage rolls, cheese straws, apple turnovers and more, this gluten-free rough puff pastry just needs a little patience and a lot of chilling. The trick is to keep the pastry as cool as possible, so maybe don't make it in the height of summer unless you're blessed with air conditioning or naturally cold hands.

Makes enough for 12 x 7.5cm sausage rolls, or 1 x 20cm pie lid

1   Place the flour, xanthan gum and salt in a large bowl and stir to combine.

2   Add the butter and use 2 dinner knives to make criss-cross cuts, chopping the butter into increasingly small pieces and working in the flour from around the sides. Keep going until the butter pieces are mostly pea-sized and well coated in the flour.

3   Gradually add the ice-cold water, stirring in each addition with a wooden spoon. Once it's all added, use your hands to bring the mixture together into a ball. Try to handle it as little as possible – you want to ensure you can still see lumps of butter throughout the pastry. At this point, if it's a warm day or the dough feels at all sticky, wrap it in clingfilm and chill for at least 20 minutes. On the other hand, if the dough feels smooth and cool, you might be able to go straight on to the next step.

4   Sprinkle a little extra flour onto a work surface and place the ball of dough in the centre. Use your hands to flatten the dough slightly and shape it into a rectangle.

5   Using a rolling pin, roll out the dough in one direction only to make a long rectangle about 1cm thick. I find the best way is to roll the dough away from you and to keep nudging the edges of the pastry with your hands to keep them reasonably straight. You should see marbled streaks of butter throughout the dough as you roll it.

6   Take the short edge that is furthest away from you and fold it towards you until it meets the centre line. Then take the edge closest to you and fold it over the doubled thickness so the pastry is in 3 layers. Wrap in clingfilm and chill for 20–30 minutes.

7   Unwrap the dough and place it on the work surface in exactly the same position as it was before. Give it a quarter-turn

TOP TIP

It can't be overstressed that you really do need to keep this pastry cold. If making it on a hot day, you might need to chill it more frequently than indicated above. If it sticks to the work surface, use a dough scraper to gently ease it off, then sprinkle the surface with a little more flour to stop it sticking again. Rolling it between clingfilm also helps to keep it cool and unsticky.

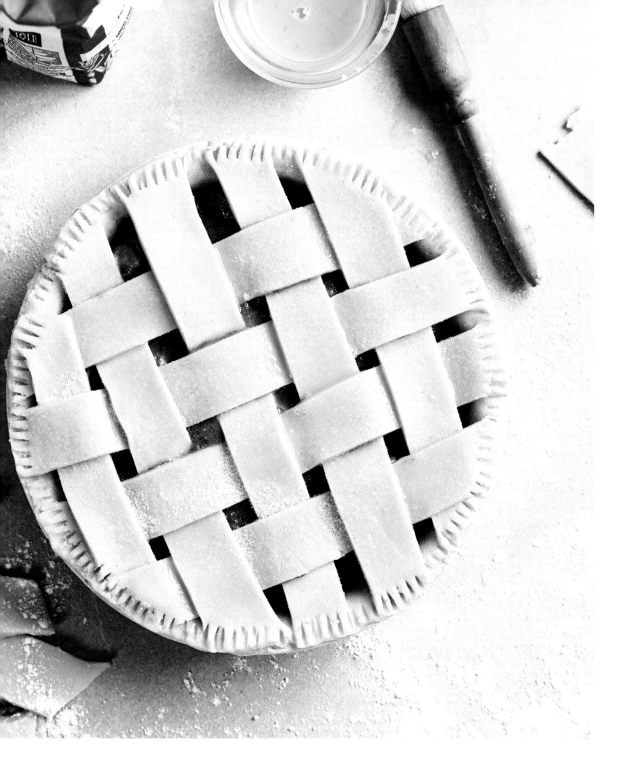

clockwise, then repeat steps 5 and 6 twice more – so a total of 3 fold-and-turns. Each time you start, place the folded dough in the same position as when you finished the last fold and give it a quarter-turn before you begin rolling.

8 Ensure you chill it for at least 20–30 minutes before rolling out for your chosen bake.

Egg Noodles

300g gluten-free white bread flour, plus extra for dusting
60g tapioca flour
1 tsp xanthan gum
6 large eggs, plus 2 egg yolks
2 tsp olive oil

Prep: **30 minutes**
Cook: **5 minutes**

DF

I don't think this recipe needs much introduction, other than to say egg noodles are probably the food I missed most when I went gluten-free. After spending 20 years pining for them, I finally made my own, realised how easy it was, and have never looked back. Trust me, if you make one thing from this book, make sure it's these noodles – you won't regret it.

Serves 4

1   Place the 2 flours in a large mixing bowl, add the xanthan gum and stir well.

2   Place the eggs and egg yolks in a small bowl or jug and whisk lightly with a fork until combined.

3   Using a wooden spoon, beat the whisked eggs a little at a time into the flour mixture. Once all added and a dough is starting to form, add the olive oil. Keep beating with a wooden spoon until the dough becomes thick and sticky. Turn it onto a piece of clingfilm, wrap tightly and leave to rest at room temperature for 15–20 minutes.

4   Lightly flour your work surface and turn the rested dough onto it. It will still be quite sticky, so lightly flour your hands, then knead the dough into a ball. Try not to add too much flour – just enough so that it forms a smooth ball

5   Flatten the ball a little with your hands, then divide into 8 equal pieces. Set 7 pieces aside, wrapped in clingfilm, to stop them from drying out.

6   Generously flour your work surface and place the unwrapped piece of dough on it. Roll it into a long rectangle about 2mm thick, turning it regularly to ensure both sides are well floured and do not stick. It should be easy to roll and handle.

7   Neaten the edges using a pizza cutter or sharp knife, then cut the rectangle into long ribbons about 2mm wide. Don't worry too much about them being exactly straight and even – a rustic appearance is fine.

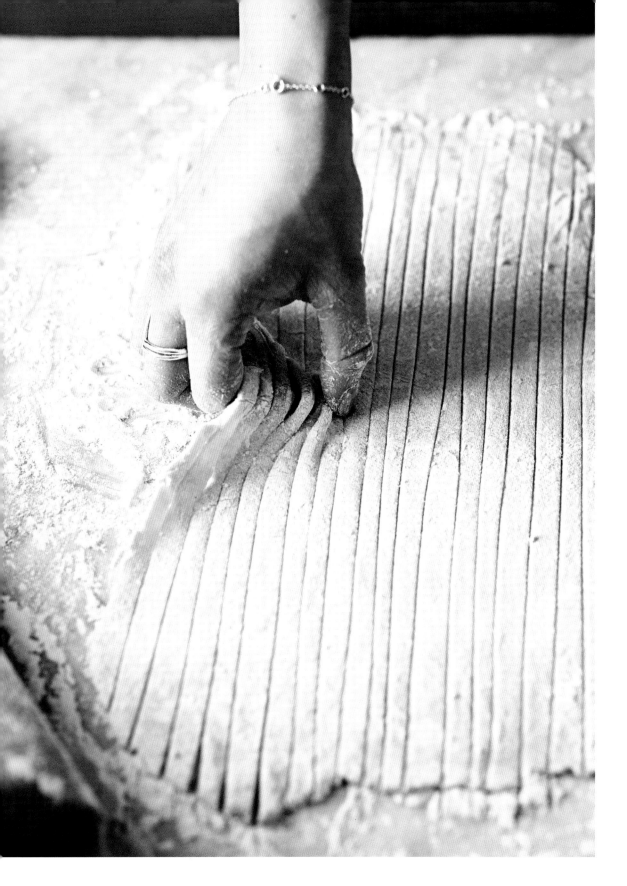

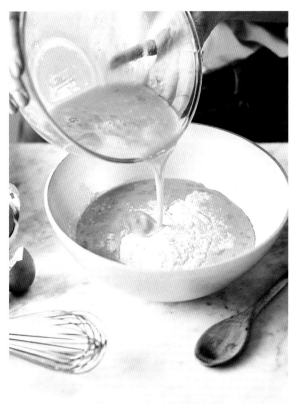

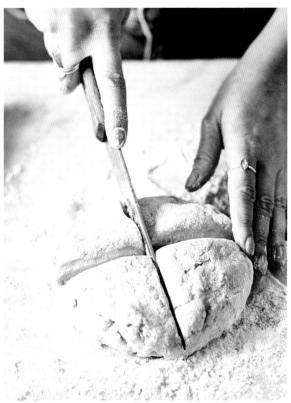

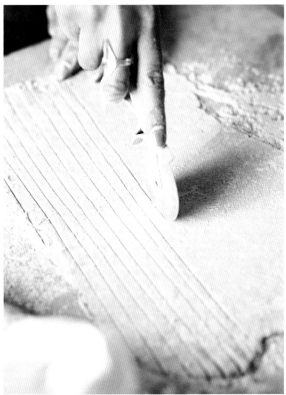

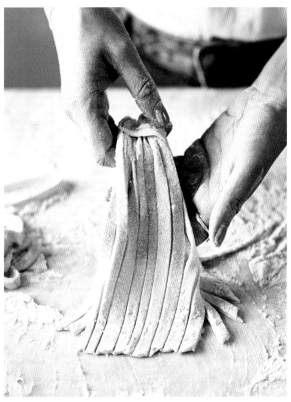

44

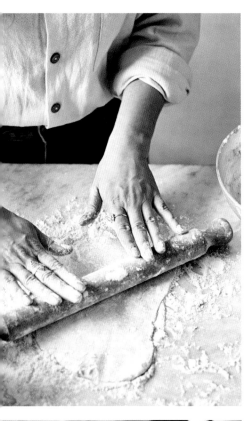

8 Gently gather up all the noodles, dust with a little extra flour, then place on a floured surface in a nest shape. Repeat steps 6, 7 and 8 with the remaining dough until you have 8 nests of noodles. Leave them to rest and dry slightly for 10–15 minutes.

9 To cook the noodles, bring a large pan of salted water to a vigorous boil and lower the nests into it. (You might need to cook them in batches so the pan is not overcrowded.) Bring back to the boil and simmer for about 2 minutes, stirring occasionally to ensure the noodles don't stick. Strain them and serve hot with your favourite Asian dishes. For inspiration, see pages 170–175.

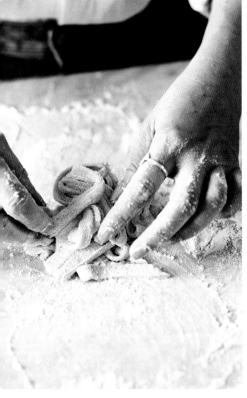

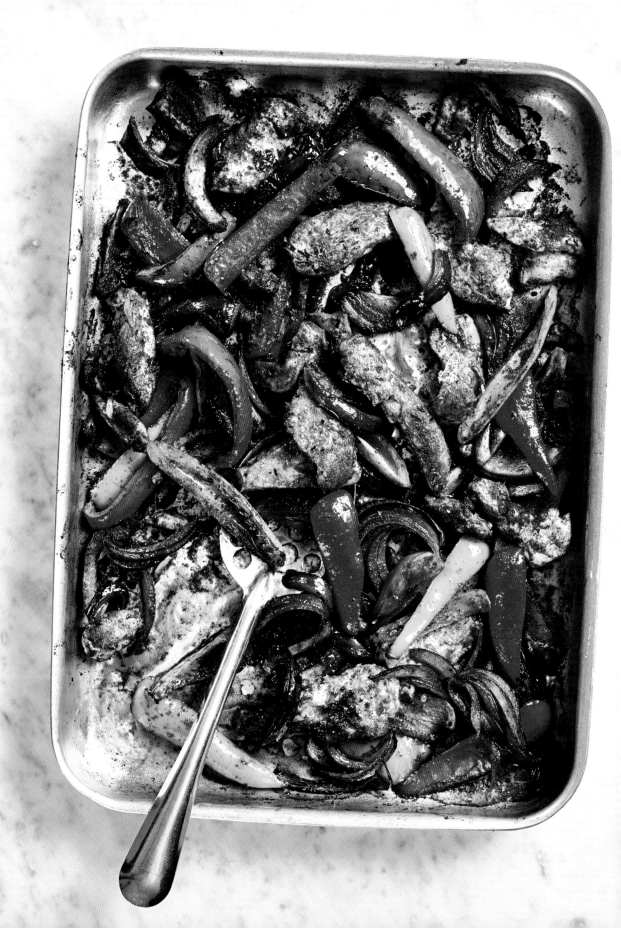

QUICK AND EASY

You know those times when you need to eat *immediately* and just don't want to spend ages in the kitchen? The quick and easy meals in this chapter can all be made in under 30 minutes and are great for anyone who is short of time – or for a self-confessed lazy person, which, let's face it, is the whole reason I eat at least three of these recipes every week...

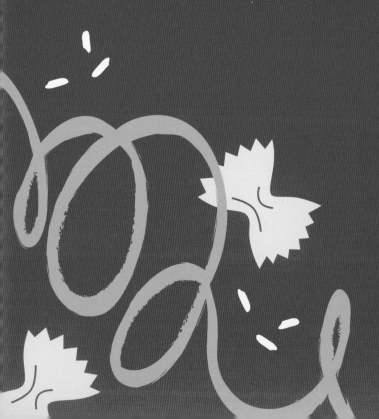

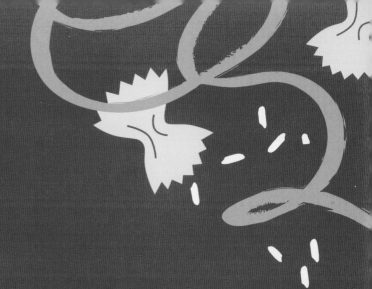

THE RECIPES

Tuna Puttanesca

400g gluten-free pasta of choice
2 tbsp olive oil
1 onion, finely chopped
3 tsp chopped garlic
2 x 400g tins chopped tomatoes
2 x 110g tins tuna, drained
½ tsp chilli flakes
160g Kalamata olives
2 tbsp capers
1 tbsp tomato purée
Fresh parsley, chopped
Parmesan cheese

Prep: **5 minutes**
Cook: **10 minutes**

EF DFO

Traditionally, puttanesca sauce is made with anchovies, but I've swapped them for tinned tuna in this effortless, store-cupboard pasta recipe. It's a great family-friendly dinner for those nights when you're in a hurry, plus you can freeze any leftover sauce for an even easier dinner on another night.

Serves 4

1 Bring a pan of salted water to the boil and cook the pasta as per the packet instructions. Make the sauce while the pasta is cooking.

2 Meanwhile, place the olive oil in a large pan over a medium heat. Once hot, add the onion and garlic and fry for 2–3 minutes, until translucent.

3 Add the tomatoes, tuna, chilli flakes, olives, capers and tomato purée and mix well. Bring to the boil, then simmer until the pasta is ready.

4 Strain the pasta, add it to the sauce and stir well to coat. Serve with a sprinkling of chopped parsley and a generous grating of Parmesan.

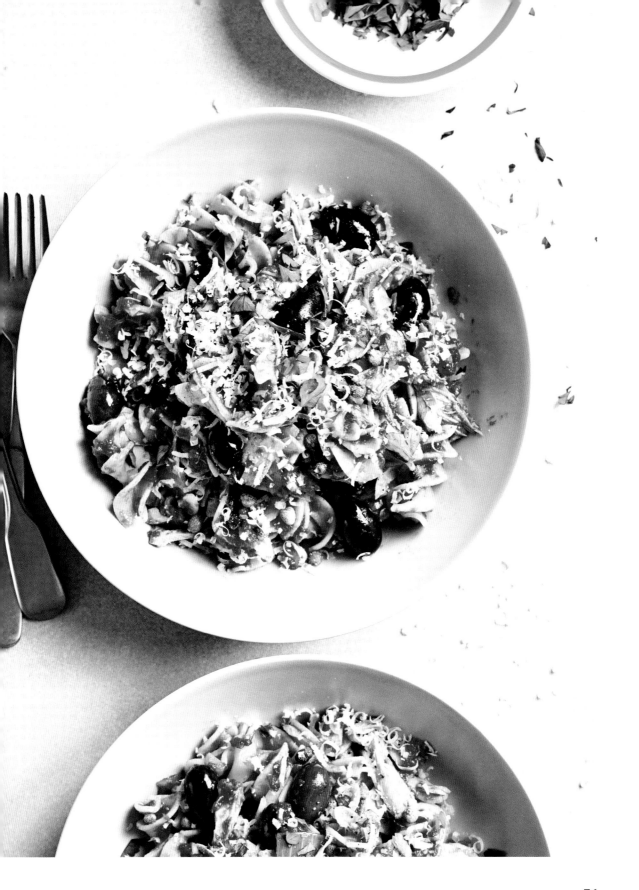

Chicken Kebabs with Easy Flatbreads

Prep: **10 minutes**
(+ up to 24 hours marinating)

Cook: **25 minutes**

 EF **DFO**

Here's a dreamy summer meal – chicken kebabs full of Mediterranean flavours served in effortless flatbreads. The simple yoghurt dough can be transformed into a gluten-free flatbread while the chicken cooks, leaving you simply to serve up the tender chicken, drizzle with the minty yoghurt and tuck in.

600g chicken thigh fillets
1 red pepper, deseeded and cut
   into 12 x 2.5cm pieces
1 red onion, cut into 8 chunks
100g Greek yoghurt or dairy-free
   alternative
1 tsp garlic powder
1 tsp dried oregano
1 tsp paprika
¼ tsp dried mint
Juice of 1 lemon
Salt and pepper
Chopped iceberg lettuce,
   to serve

For the flatbreads
200g gluten-free plain flour
2 tsp baking powder
200g Greek yoghurt or dairy-free
   alternative
1 tsp salt
2 tsp dried oregano

For the yoghurt drizzle
100g Greek yoghurt or dairy-free
   alternative
Juice of 1 lemon
1 tsp garlic granules
½ tsp dried mint

Serves 4 _____

1   Cut the chicken into 5cm chunks.

2   Put the yoghurt in a large bowl with the garlic powder, oregano, paprika, mint, lemon juice, a generous seasoning of salt and pepper and mix well. Add the chicken to the bowl, mixing until it is completely coated. Leave to marinate in the fridge for at least 1 hour, but it's even better if left overnight.

3   Preheat the oven to 220ºC/Fan 200ºC/Gas Mark 7.

4   Take 4 skewers and thread with the chicken pieces, interspersed with the pepper and red onion chunks. Lie the skewers across a roasting tray so that the ends rest on the rim and the chicken is suspended over the tray. Place in the oven for 25 minutes, rotating the skewers after 10–15 minutes so they cook evenly.

5   Meanwhile, place the flatbread ingredients in a large bowl and mix together until a sticky dough forms. Divide the dough into 4 equal pieces and roll each one into a ball. Place a ball of dough between 2 sheets of baking paper and use a rolling pin to roll into a circle about 4mm thick.

6   Place a large, dry frying pan over a high heat. When hot, peel the top layer of paper off the dough circle, then use the bottom paper to flip the circle into the pan. Peel off the paper and lower the heat to medium. Fry the flatbread on

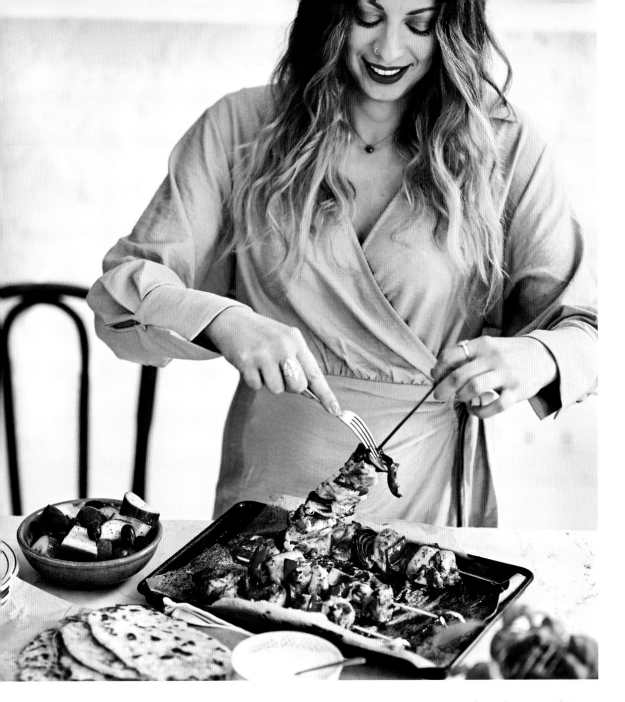

TOP TIP ▶▶▶▶

To be dairy free, the yoghurt in this recipe can easily be replaced with a dairy-free alternative. I find coconut yoghurt makes the best flatbreads.

each side for 2 minutes, then remove from the pan and wrap in foil to keep warm while you repeat steps 7 and 8 to make 4 flatbreads in all.

7 Mix the yoghurt drizzle ingredients together in a bowl.

8 When the chicken is done, place some lettuce in the centre of each flatbread, then use a fork to ease the chicken and veg off the skewers and onto the lettuce. Drizzle with the yoghurt dressing and serve straight away.

Butter, Sage & Pancetta Gnocchi

1 quantity gluten-free gnocchi (see page 34)
100g unsalted butter

Small handful of sage leaves
250g pancetta cubes
300g spinach leaves

Cook: **10 minutes**

EF

With only five ingredients and ready in ten minutes, this could possibly be the easiest meal ever. I absolutely love the simple pairing of sage and butter, but add the salty element of pancetta and it's even better. For a vegetarian version, simply omit the pancetta and add a sprinkling of salt.

Serves 4

1 Bring a large pan of salted water to the boil.

2 Meanwhile, melt the butter in a large frying pan over a low heat. Add the sage leaves and fry for 1–2 minutes, until crispy. Remove with a slotted spoon and set to one side.

3 Add the pancetta to the frying pan and fry for 5 minutes.

4 Meanwhile, add the gnocchi to the boiling water and cook for 3 minutes, until they start to rise to the surface. Drain well, reserving 2 tablespoons of the cooking water.

5 Once the pancetta is crispy, add the spinach and fry for another minute, until the leaves have wilted.

6 Add the drained gnocchi, the reserved cooking water and most of the sage leaves. Mix well, then serve straight away, sprinkling the remaining sage leaves on top.

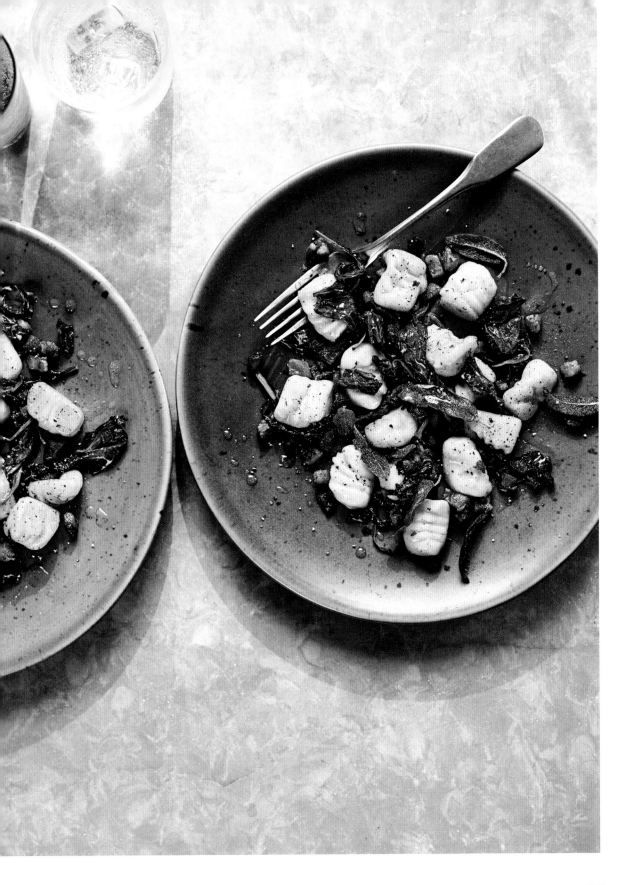

Chicken Fajita Traybake

Prep: **10 minutes**
Cook: **20 minutes**

Sizzling fajitas are traditionally made in a pan, but turning them into a traybake takes out all the effort of standing over a hot stove. This is a great meal for families or groups of friends to tuck into, and any leftovers make an absolutely banging salad, sandwich or wrap for lunch the next day. If you like things super fiery, try adding some chopped jalapeños to the salsa and swap the mild chilli powder for hot.

3 mixed peppers, deseeded and sliced into 2cm strips
1 large red onion, sliced
2 large chicken breasts, sliced into 2cm strips
2 tbsp vegetable oil
12 gluten-free Tortilla Wraps (see page 37)

For the fajita spice mix
2 tsp mild chilli powder
2 tsp paprika
½ tsp ground cumin
1 tsp garlic granules
½ tsp cayenne pepper
½ tsp onion salt
1 tsp oregano
Salt and pepper

For the tomato salsa
150g cherry tomatoes, quartered
1 small white onion, finely chopped
Juice of 1 lime
Handful of fresh coriander, chopped

To serve
1 iceberg lettuce, shredded
Grated cheese (optional)

Serves 4

1 Preheat the oven to 220ºC/Fan 200ºC/Gas Mark 7.

2 Mix all the fajita spices together in a small dish, along with a generous seasoning of salt and pepper.

3 Add the sliced vegetables and chicken strips to a large bowl and pour over the oil. Mix well, then sprinkle over the spices and mix again until everything is evenly coated.

4 Empty the chicken bowl into a large non-stick roasting tray and spread out evenly. (You can use 2 trays if you only have small ones.)

5 Place in the oven for 10 minutes, then use a spoon to turn the veg and chicken so they cook evenly. Return to the oven for another 10 minutes.

6 Wrap the tortillas in foil and place them on the shelf underneath the chicken for the remaining cooking time.

7 Make the salsa by combining the tomatoes, onion, lime juice and three-quarters of the chopped coriander in a small bowl. Set to one side.

8 When the cooking time is up, remove the tray and tortilla wraps from the oven. Sprinkle the remaining coriander over the chicken and veg, then place the tray on the table along with the hot wraps, shredded lettuce and grated cheese, if using. Invite hungry diners to heap their wraps with the fillings and add a smothering of salsa.

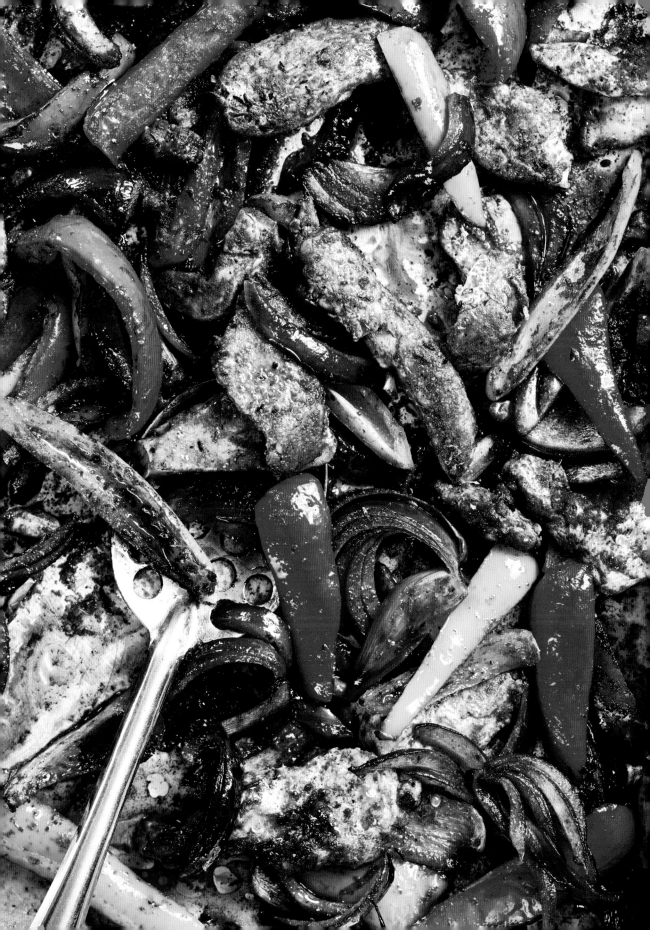

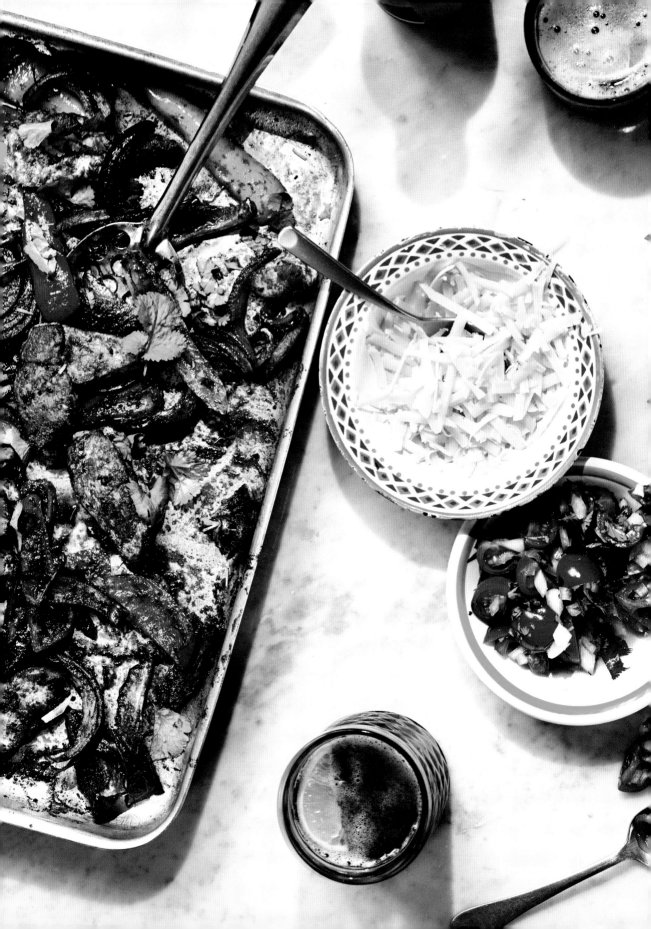

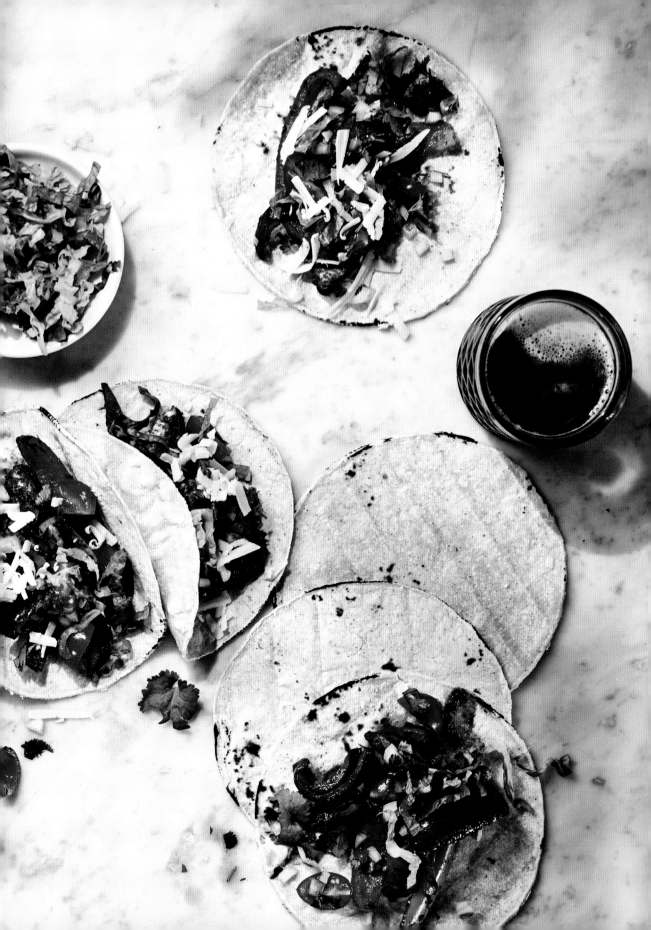

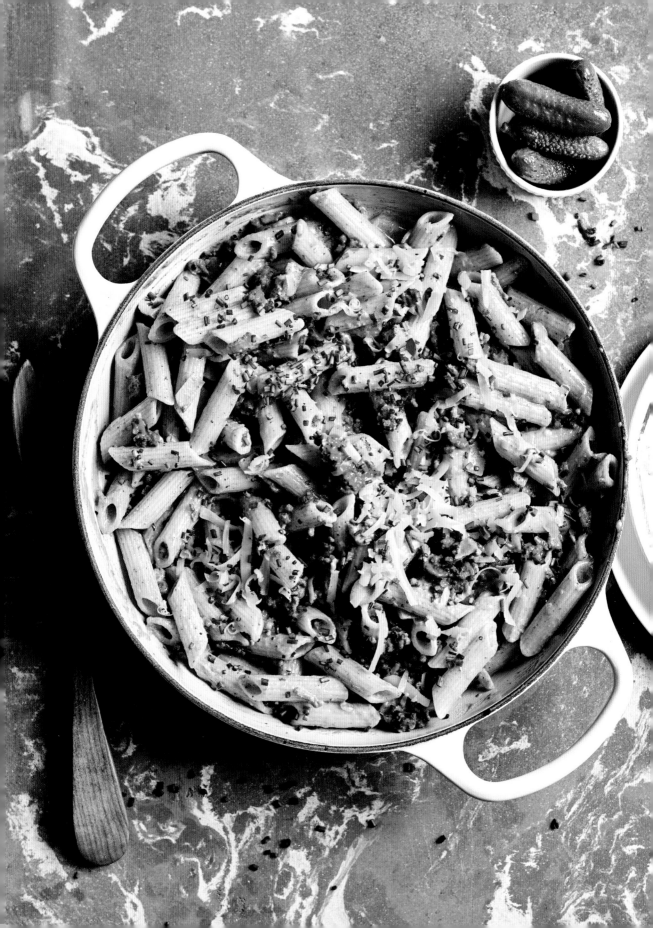

Cheeseburger Pasta

400g gluten-free pasta
1 tbsp olive oil
500g lean beef mince
1 small onion, finely diced
1 tsp garlic paste, or 1 garlic
  clove, crushed
1 tsp paprika

100g full-fat cream cheese
150g Red Leicester cheese,
  grated, plus extra to serve
275ml gluten-free vegetable
  stock
Salt and pepper
Chopped chives, to serve

Prep: **5 minutes**
(+ 25 minutes if baking)

Cook: **10 minutes**

EF

Imagine if a cheeseburger and a bowl of mac and cheese had a gluten-free baby and you're pretty much on track for the wicked deliciousness that is this Cheeseburger Pasta. To those new to the concept, it's a gorgeously creamy, cheesy pasta sauce mixed with beef mince to create the hybrid pasta of dreams. What makes this dish even more decadent? Only the fact you can be slobbing on the sofa scoffing a bowl of it in less than 15 minutes.

Serves 4

1   Bring a large pan of generously salted water to the boil. Add the pasta and cook as per the packet instructions.

2   Meanwhile, warm the oil in a large, heavy-based pan over a medium-high heat. Once hot, add the mince, onion, garlic and paprika, stir together and fry until the beef has browned, the onions have softened, and any excess liquid from the meat has boiled off – this will take about 5–7 minutes.

3   Turn the heat down to medium-low and add the cream cheese and Red Leicester to the beef mixture. Pour in the vegetable stock, then stir and cook the mixture until the cheese has melted and formed a thick, creamy sauce. Leave to simmer gently until the pasta is ready.

4   Once the pasta is cooked, add 1–2 tablespoons of the cooking water to the sauce, depending how thick you want it.

5   Drain the pasta, add to the sauce and stir well. Sprinkle over some extra grated cheese and chopped chives and serve straight away, or place under the grill to melt the cheese. You could even bake it in the oven at 200ºC/Fan 180ºC/Gas Mark 6 for a further 15 minutes or so if you want a crispy cheese topping and a dish that is more like a cheeseburger pasta bake.

TOP TIP

I know gherkins divide the nation, but if you're a fan, you can finish this dish off beautifully with a sprinkling of chopped gherkins for the full cheeseburger experience.

Cheat's Chilaquiles

Prep: **5 minutes**
Cook: **15 minutes**

This simple and tasty Mexican breakfast is usually made using stale tortilla wraps, which are cut into triangles and deep-fried. While you're welcome to try this if you like, my cheat's version uses gluten-free corn tortilla chips, and the dish is not only great, but the perfect hangover cure! Just make sure the tortilla chips you buy are actually gluten free, as not all brands are.

1 red onion, roughly chopped
2 green chillies, deseeded
4 tsp chopped garlic
2 x 400g tins chopped tomatoes
200ml gluten-free vegetable stock
2–3 tbsp vegetable oil
4 large eggs
400g plain or salted gluten-free corn tortilla chips
100g feta cheese
Handful of fresh coriander, chopped

Serves 4

1 Place the onion, chillies, garlic, tomatoes and vegetable stock in the bowl of a food processor and blitz to make a sauce. Pour into a frying pan, bring to the boil, then simmer for 7–8 minutes, until thickened.

2 Meanwhile, heat the oil in a separate frying pan and fry the eggs to your liking – I prefer them to have a runny yolk for this recipe, but go with your personal preference.

3 Once the eggs are done and the sauce has thickened, remove the eggs from the heat. Add the tortilla chips to the sauce, stir well so they are evenly coated, then take off the heat.

4 Divide the tortilla chip sauce equally between 4 bowls, then sit a fried egg on top of each one. Crumble the feta over the top and sprinkle with chopped coriander to finish.

TOP TIP

Feel free to add some sliced, fresh red chilli on top of the chilaquiles for extra zing. Creamy chunks of avocado are also a great addition.

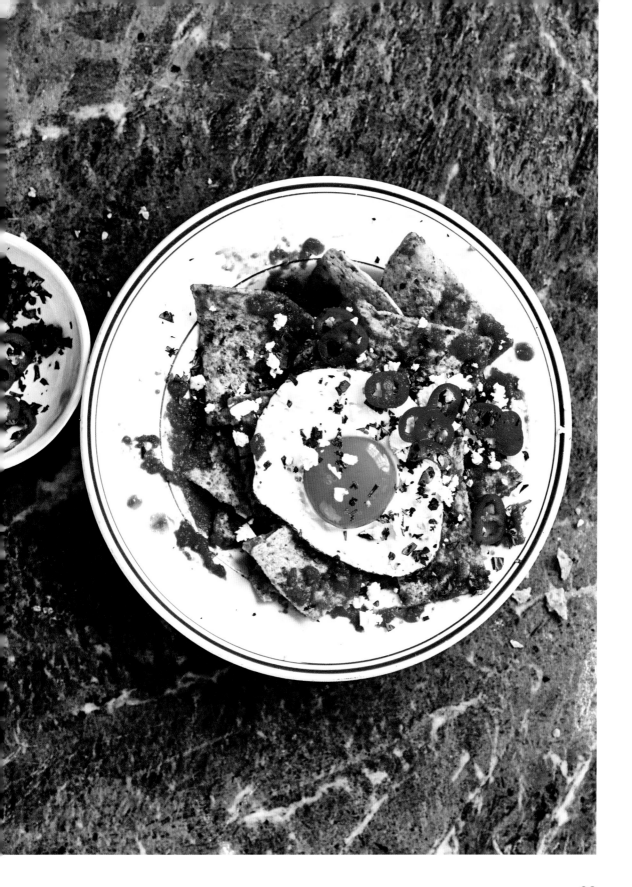

Cajun Chicken Burgers

2 chicken breasts
8 rashers smoked streaky bacon
1–2 tbsp olive oil
4 gluten-free burger buns
4 slices Gouda cheese
4 tsp mayonnaise
1 avocado, peeled and sliced
2 tomatoes, thinly sliced

For the spice mix
2 tbsp cornflour
2 tsp onion salt
2 tsp garlic granules
2 tsp smoked paprika
2 tsp cayenne pepper
2 tsp ground cumin
2 tsp dried oregano
Salt and pepper

Prep: **10 minutes**
Cook: **10 minutes**

These easy Cajun chicken burgers are big on flavours but can be thrown together really fast. If you want to save on washing up, you can always fry the bacon in the same pan as the chicken, but nothing beats crispy grilled bacon in my eyes. Any leftover chicken is great in a salad or gluten-free wrap for lunch the next day.

Serves 4

1 Place the spice mix ingredients on a plate, season well with salt and pepper and mix thoroughly.

2 Cut the chicken breasts in half lengthways and place them between 2 sheets of clingfilm. Bash with a rolling pin to flatten them, then remove the film.

3 Dip each chicken piece in the spice mix, coating them completely.

4 Preheat the grill to medium-high and grill the bacon for 2 minutes on each side, until crispy. (Grill for a little longer if you like it super-crispy.)

5 Meanwhile, add the oil to a frying pan over a medium-high heat. Once hot, fry the chicken pieces for 2–3 minutes on each side, until cooked through.

6 Cut the burger buns in half and place under the grill for a minute to toast lightly. Add a cheese slice to one half of each bun and grill for another 30–60 seconds, until the cheese has melted.

7 To construct each burger, slather the mayo on the bottom half of a burger bun. Add a piece of chicken, followed by 2 bacon rashers, a quarter of the avocado and a few tomato slices. Top with the cheesy burger bun.

 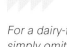

TOP TIP

For a dairy-free option, simply omit the Gouda slices or replace them with your favourite dairy-free cheese instead.

64

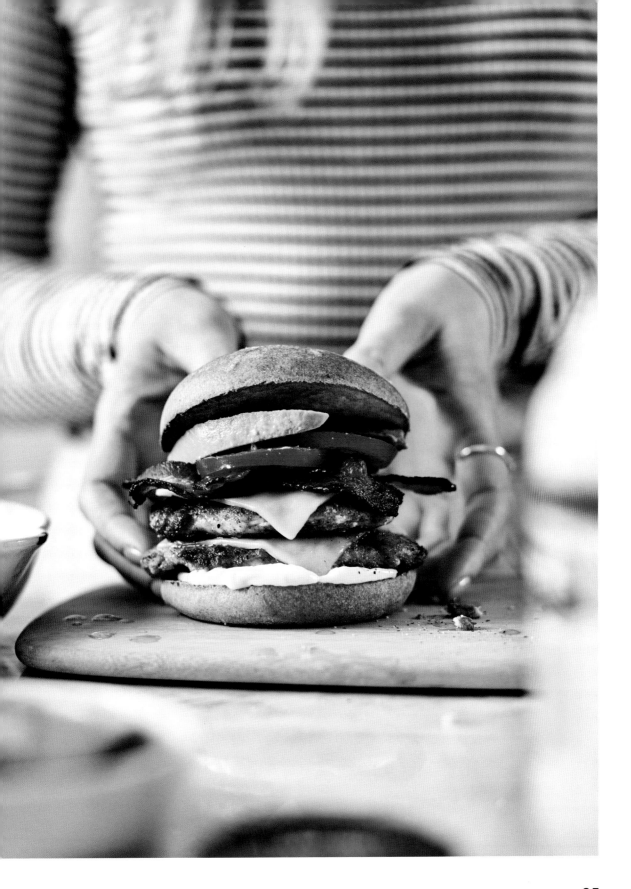

Mediterranean Quesadillas

4 gluten-free Tortilla Wraps (see page 37)
300g cooked chicken, shredded or thinly sliced
100g green olives, sliced
12 sun-dried tomatoes, roughly chopped
4 handfuls of baby spinach leaves (about 60g)
125g mozzarella cheese or dairy-free alternative, sliced

Prep: **5 minutes**
Cook: **5 minutes**

I do love a bit of fusion when it comes to food, so turning a Mexican dish into a Mediterranean-style lunch is right up my street. Quesadillas are always a really quick and easy option for a light meal, and of course you can always mix the fillings up however you like. I usually serve one of these per person, or two if a more substantial meal is needed.

Serves 4

1   Lay out the wraps and cover half of each one with the cooked chicken. Scatter the olives and sun-dried tomatoes on top, then add the spinach leaves. Top with slices of the mozzarella.

2   Fold the empty half of each wrap over the fillings and press down firmly.

3   Place a large frying pan over a medium-high heat. Once hot, add the quesadillas 1 or 2 at a time, depending how big the pan is, and cook for 2 minutes on each side. Cook for another 2 minutes, until the cheese has melted.

4   Remove from the pan, cut in half and serve. If you're cooking these in batches, you can keep them in a warm oven while you cook the rest.

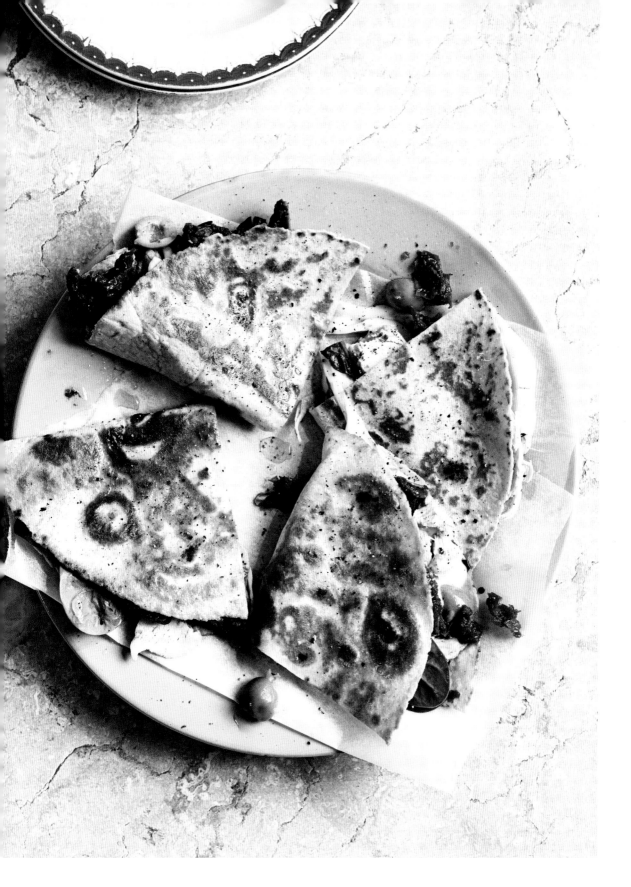

Chorizo & Cod Rice Pan

Prep: **5 minutes**
Cook: **25 minutes**

EF **DF**

1 tbsp olive oil
150g chorizo, diced
1 red onion, finely chopped
2 tsp chopped garlic
250g roasted red peppers from
  a jar, chopped
1 tsp dried oregano
1 tsp smoked paprika

200g uncooked basmati rice
1 x 400g tin of chickpeas,
  drained
500ml gluten-free vegetable
  stock
4 cod fillets, about 360g in total
Handful of fresh parsley,
  chopped

Whenever I'm in a hurry, this is often my go-to meal. Not only is it ready in half an hour, it's also naturally gluten free and cooks all in one pan, meaning I can leave it simmering while I get on with other important things, such as scrolling through funny dog videos on my phone. The sweet red peppers and fiery chorizo go so well with the flaky cod, and it's a great dish to have cold in a lunchbox the next day too.

Serves 4

1 Place the olive oil in a large pan over a medium heat. When hot, add the chorizo, onion, garlic and red peppers. Fry for 4–5 minutes, until the onions are translucent.

2 Add the oregano, smoked paprika, rice and chickpeas to the pan and mix well.

3 Pour in the stock, stir well and cover with a lid. Turn the heat right down and simmer for 10 minutes without removing the lid.

4 Meanwhile, cut each cod fillet in half.

5 Uncover the pan and nestle the cod pieces down into the rice mixture. Replace the lid and cook for another 5–10 minutes, until the fish is cooked through and flaky.

6 Remove from the heat, sprinkle with the chopped parsley and serve.

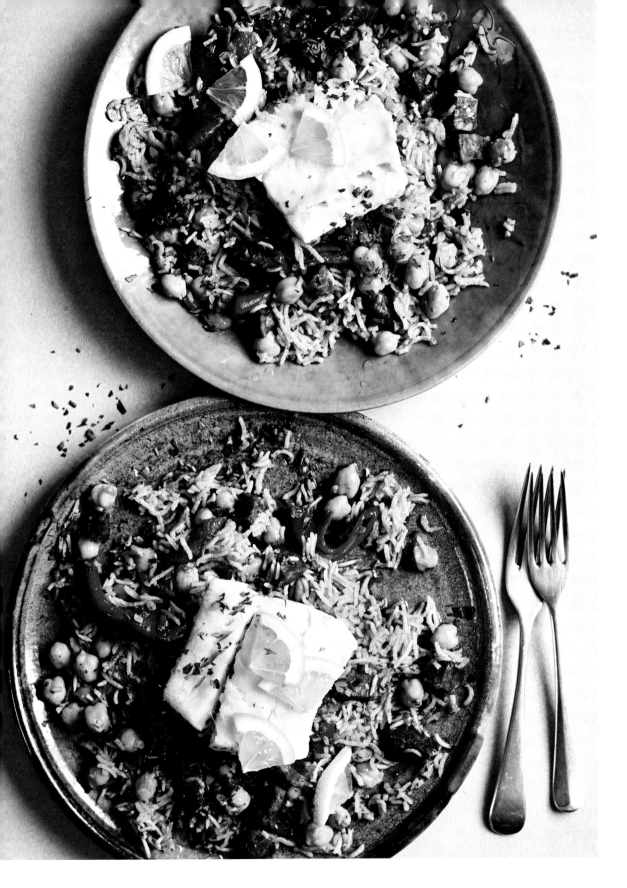

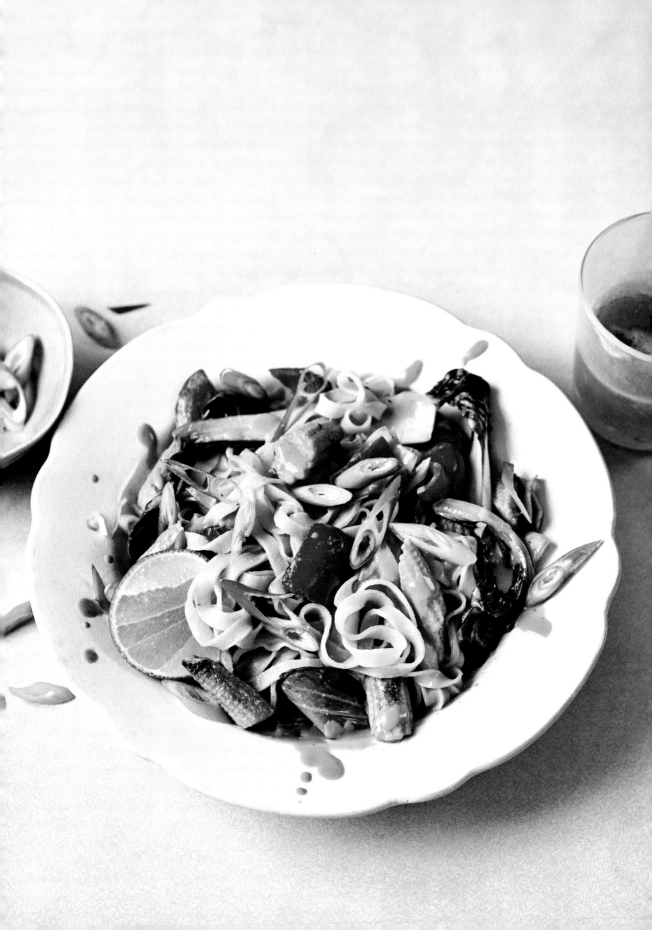

Thai Peanut Noodles

Prep: **5 minutes**
Cook: **10 minutes**

 EF DF   V

These nutty noodles are great for when you need a simple yet nourishing meal. The dish is packed with vegetables and really quick to throw together – plus I love the fiery little kick from using sriracha in the sauce.

1 tbsp sesame oil
200g pak choi, sliced
1 red pepper, deseeded and chopped into chunks
80g baby corn, chopped into chunks
3 spring onions, chopped
225g flat rice noodles

Lime wedges, to serve

For the sauce
100g peanut butter
2 tbsp tamari sauce
1 tbsp sriracha sauce
Juice of 1 lime

Serves 4 _____

1   Combine the sauce ingredients in a bowl and set to one side.

2   Place the sesame oil in a wok over a high heat. Once hot, add the vegetables, reserving a handful of spring onions for serving, and stir-fry for 3–4 minutes.

3   Cook the noodles as per the packet instructions. When ready, stir 4 tablespoons of the cooking water into the sauce, then drain the noodles and rinse in cold water.

4   Add the noodles to the wok, then pour in the sauce. Stir-fry for 1–2 minutes, until the sauce is mixed through.

5   Serve sprinkled with the reserved spring onions and a lime wedge on the side.

Fish Fingers

Prep: **10 minutes**
Cook: **10 minutes**

DF

400g skinless cod fillets
2 tbsp gluten-free plain flour
100g gluten-free Panko
   Breadcrumbs (see page 38)
1 large egg
Vegetable oil, for frying
Salt and pepper

For the peas
160g frozen peas
Juice of ½ lemon
½ tsp chilli flakes

For the tartare sauce
4 tbsp mayonnaise
6 gherkin slices, finely chopped
2 tsp capers, finely chopped

Fish fingers are such a homely treat, and you can't beat serving them up with homemade tartare sauce and a good dollop of lemony mashed peas. These rustic fingers are much nicer than shop-bought ones, and freeze well too. They also make a great butty when slapped between two thick slices of gluten-free bread.

Serves 4

1. Use kitchen paper to pat any moisture off the fish, then cut the fillets into strips 2cm wide.

2. Place the flour on a plate and mix in a generous seasoning of salt and pepper.

3. Place the panko breadcrumbs on a separate plate.

4. Beat the egg and add it to a third plate.

5. Take a piece of the fish and coat it first in the flour, then in the egg and finally in the breadcrumbs, pressing them in to ensure the coating is complete. Set to one side and repeat with all the remaining fish.

6. Pour a 5mm depth of oil into a frying pan and place over a medium heat. Once hot, add the fish pieces in batches and fry for 2–3 minutes each side, until golden brown. Transfer to a plate lined with kitchen paper and keep warm.

7. Meanwhile, place the peas and 1 tablespoon water in a heatproof bowl, cover with a plate and microwave for 2–3 minutes. When cooked, drain the peas and transfer them to a food processor with the lemon juice, chilli flakes and salt and pepper. Blitz to a coarse purée.

8. Make the tartare sauce by combining all the ingredients for it in a bowl.

9. Serve the fish fingers with the peas, a dollop of tartare sauce and a green salad.

TOP TIP

For a lower-fat version of these fish fingers, you can bake them in the oven at 200ºC/Fan 180ºC/Gas Mark 6 for 15–20 minutes instead of frying in oil. They don't become as crunchy and golden as fried ones, but they're just as tasty.

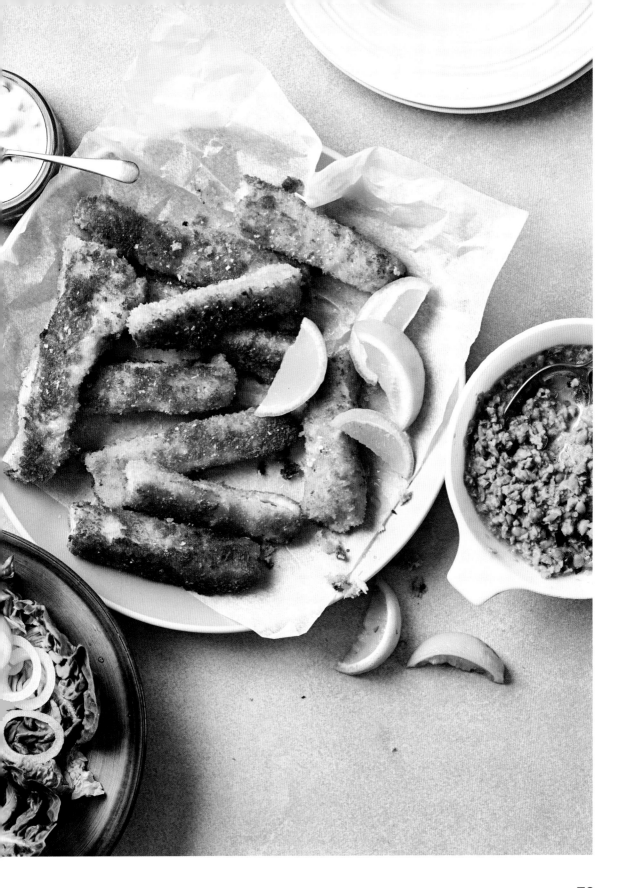

'Ugly' Pot Noodles

Prep: **2 minutes**
Cook: **3 minutes**

You know how sometimes you make a meal that tastes good, but visually just doesn't quite cut it? Meet my ugly pot noodles. They may not be the most Insta-worthy dish, but damn, do they taste good! What's more, they take only five minutes to throw together and are the most convenient packed lunch. All you have to do is assemble them at home in a lunchbox, then add hot water and microwave at work. No microwave? No problem! Make a batch and pack them in a vacuum flask to take with you wherever you're heading. Just don't forget cutlery...

1 gluten-free vermicelli rice noodle nest
1 spring onion, chopped
50g carrot, grated
25g fresh or frozen peas
50g cooked chicken, shredded
½ gluten-free chicken stock cube
2 tsp tamari sauce
1 tsp sriracha sauce
1 tsp miso paste
300ml boiling water

Serves 1

1   Place the rice noodles in a heatproof container or bowl, and sit the spring onion, carrot, peas and chicken on top.

2   Crumble in the chicken stock cube, then add the tamari, sriracha and miso paste.

3   When you're ready to eat, pour in 300ml boiling water and microwave on full power for 2–3 minutes, until the noodles have cooked. Stir well and serve straight away.

TOP TIP

For a veggie version, omit the chicken and use a vegetable stock cube. You could also add 1 teaspoon curry powder or Thai curry paste for a different flavour. Other vegetables that work well include sweetcorn, finely chopped peppers and baby spinach leaves.

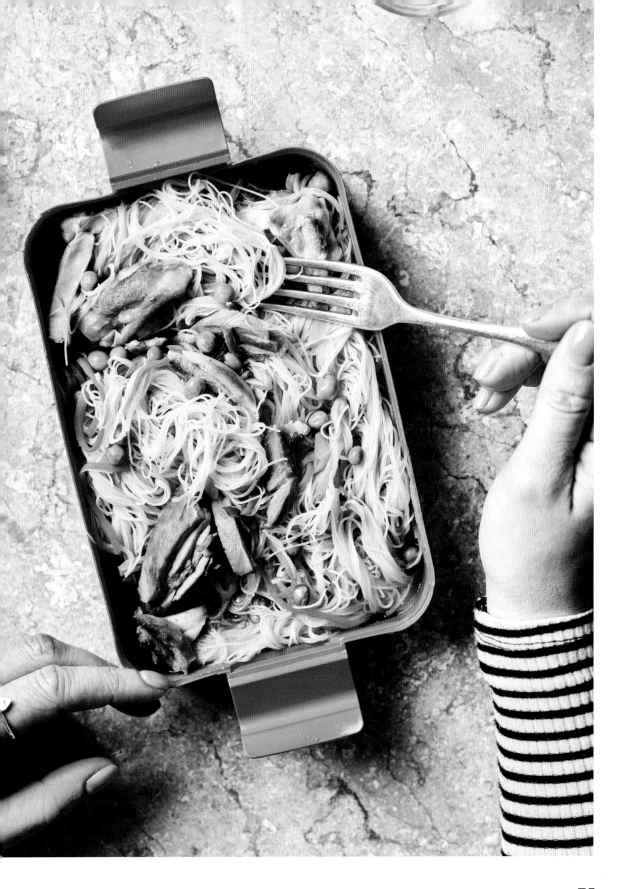

Chickpea, Quinoa & Halloumi Salad

1 tbsp olive oil
225g halloumi cheese, cut into 1–2cm cubes
1 x 250g pouch cooked quinoa
1 red onion, chopped
130g sun-dried tomatoes
40g rocket leaves
75g chopped walnuts
1 x 400g tin chickpeas, drained

For the dressing
1 tbsp olive oil
1 tbsp balsamic vinegar
1 tbsp maple syrup

Prep: **5 minutes**
Cook: **5 minutes**

I do sometimes miss having grains in my salads, but quinoa provides the perfect alternative to them. Not only is it fun to say – you pronounce it 'keen-wah', daaarling – but this South American delight is a protein-packed seed that fills the couscous-shaped hole in my life. My best friend Lauren taught me the three-ingredient dressing, and I became so obsessed that I poured it over pretty much every meal I had for a whole summer. This salad is a great summer main course or gluten-free side for a barbecue.

Serves 2 as a main, 4 as a side

1 Place the oil in a frying pan over a medium-high heat. Once hot, fry the halloumi cubes, stirring frequently, until they start to brown on each side.

2 Meanwhile, heat the quinoa as per the packet instructions.

3 Place the dressing ingredients in a small tub or jar, tighten the lid and shake well to mix.

4 Put all the remaining salad ingredients into a large serving bowl, add the quinoa and halloumi, then pour over the dressing. Toss well to combine and serve straight away.

TOP TIP

For a dairy-free option, simply omit the halloumi or replace with a vegan version.

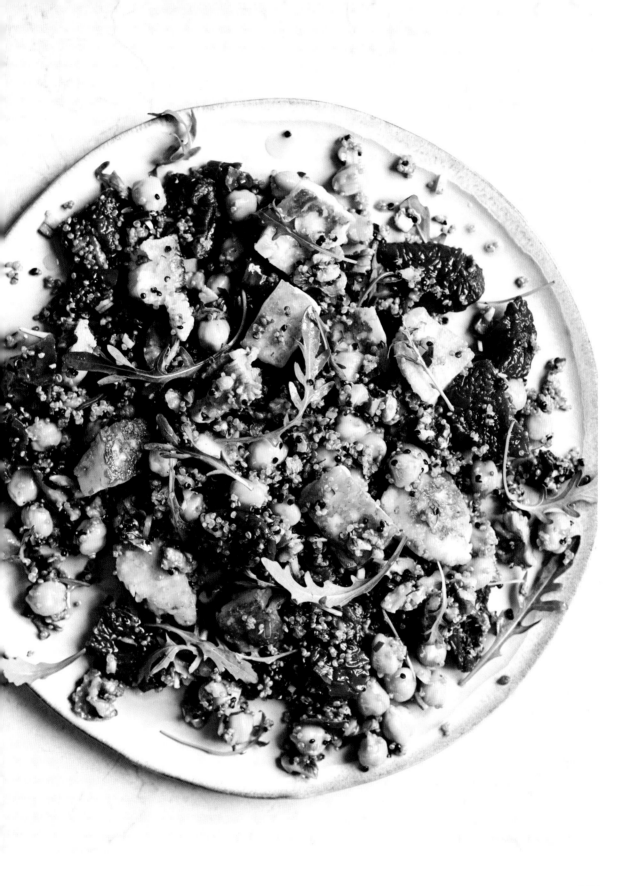

Chickpea, Sweetcorn & Feta Fritters

Prep: **5 minutes**
Cook: **15 minutes**

1 x 400g tin chickpeas
200g tinned sweetcorn
2 spring onions, chopped
1 red chilli, deseeded and chopped
1 tsp chopped garlic
40g gluten-free plain flour
1 tsp smoked paprika
150g feta cheese
1–2 tbsp olive oil
Salt and pepper
Sweet chilli sauce, to serve

With a golden crunch on the outside and bursts of feta and chilli inside, these fritters are the perfect light meal. I love to serve them hot with a fresh green salad and a bowl of sweet chilli sauce for dipping. They're also delicious when cold, so are great in lunchboxes; or try combining them with salad ingredients in one of my gluten-free tortilla wraps (see page 37).

Serves 4

1 Drain the chickpeas, reserving the liquid in a bowl. Place the chickpeas in a food processor with 150g of the sweetcorn, the spring onions, chilli, garlic, flour and smoked paprika. Pulse until the mixture is combined – it doesn't need to be completely smooth.

2 Add 1–2 tablespoons of the reserved chickpea liquid and blitz again to loosen the mixture slightly.

3 Remove the bowl from the processor. Add the remaining sweetcorn, crumble in the feta, season generously with salt and pepper and stir to combine.

4 Divide the mixture into 8 equal portions; you might want to weigh the mixture to do this accurately.

5 Using wet hands, shape each portion into a ball, then flatten into a patty about 2–3cm thick.

6 Place the olive oil in a large frying pan over a medium heat. Once hot, add 3–4 of the patties, ensuring you have space between them, and fry for 3–4 minutes, until browned on one side. Gently flip and fry for another 3–4 minutes. Transfer to a plate, cover with foil and keep warm in a low oven.

7 Fry the other patties in the same way, adding a little extra olive oil if needed. Once they are all cooked, serve hot with salad and sweet chilli sauce for dipping.

TOP TIP

If you want to make these fritters dairy-free or vegan, simply omit the feta completely, or replace it with a vegan feta alternative.

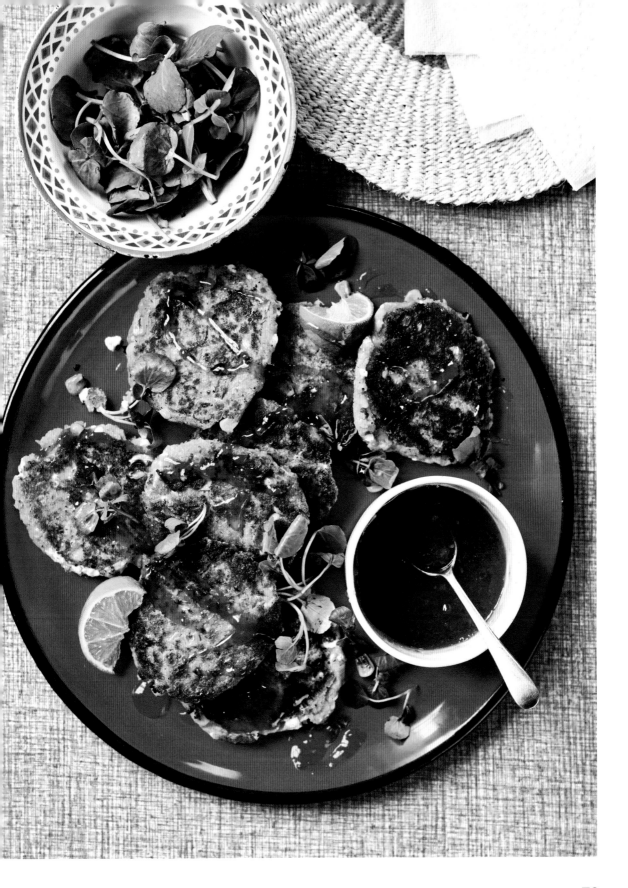

Chorizo Carbonara

400g gluten-free spaghetti
Olive oil
1 chorizo ring, about 225g
4 large eggs

100g pecorino cheese, grated,
plus extra for sprinkling
Black pepper

Prep: **5 minutes**
Cook: **10 minutes**

I love a traditional carbonara, but switching the pancetta for chorizo gives it a spicy twist. This simple and tasty meal is ready in less than 15 minutes, and it's always my go-to on nights when I get home late, as there is nearly always chorizo in the fridge. You could try adding a few spinach leaves or peas if you like, but sometimes simplicity is best.

Serves 4

1   Bring a large pan of salted water to the boil, then add a drop of olive oil followed by the spaghetti. Cook as per the packet instructions, until al dente.

2   Meanwhile, peel the chorizo and roughly chop or crumble the meat into small pieces. Add to a dry pan over a medium heat and fry for 3–4 minutes, until starting to crisp up. The oil that seeps out of the chorizo should be enough without adding any extra. Turn the heat off once crispy, but leave in the pan.

3   Place the eggs and pecorino in a bowl, add a good twist of black pepper and beat together.

4   When the spaghetti has cooked, don't drain it – use tongs to transfer it to the chorizo pan. Any water still clinging to it will help to emulsify the sauce. Add an extra tablespoon of the pasta water, then pour in the egg mixture and use the tongs to mix together. Don't turn on the heat or you'll scramble the eggs.

5   Serve the spaghetti in bowls, sprinkling them with extra pecorino and a twist of black pepper.

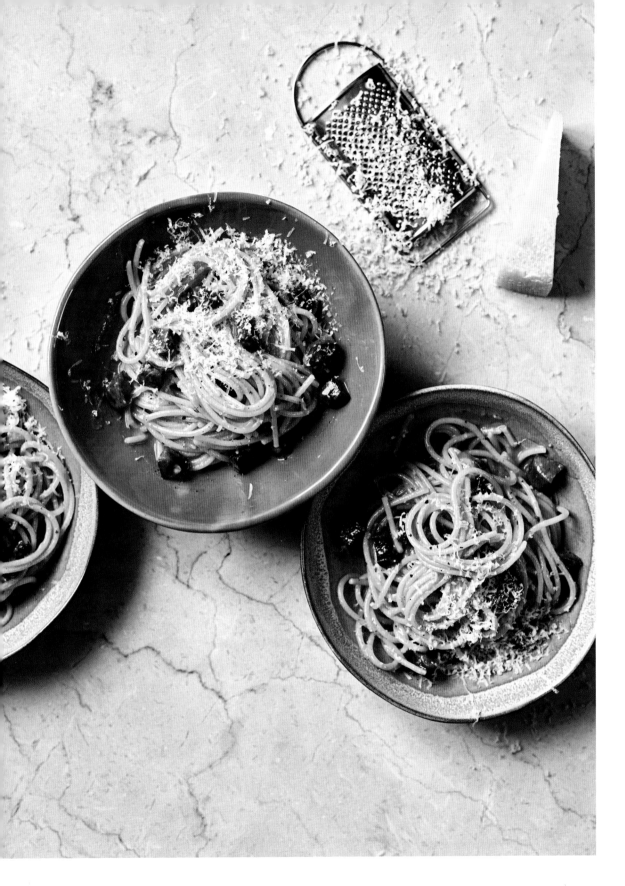

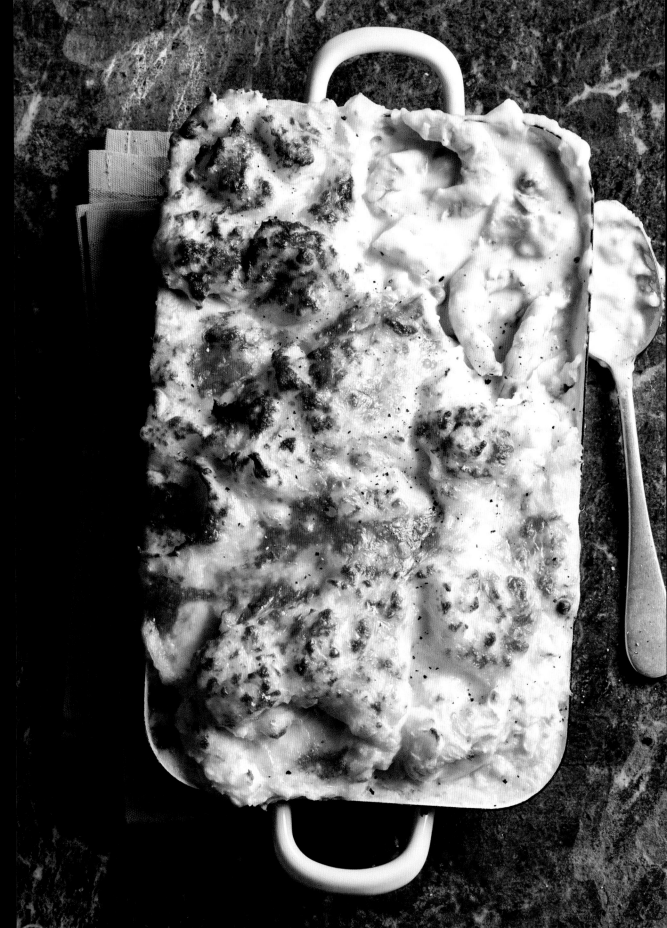

BATCH-COOK HEROES

The secret to saving time, money and effort lies in this chapter. As the old saying goes, 'Cook once, eat twice'. Your freezer is about to become your best friend here because storing extra portions means you'll always have an easy microwave dinner at hand for those nights when you just can't be bothered to cook. Trust me, I should know – I have those nights often. Also, any leftovers make for excellent, easy-to-reheat lunches. The recipes here serve four, but the amounts listed can be doubled or even trebled, depending on the size of your household, or the amount you want to stash in the freezer for later.

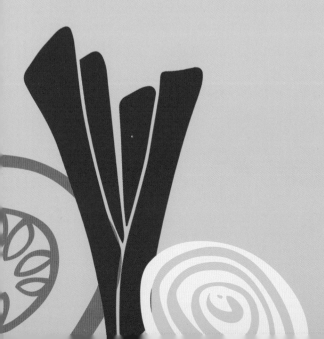

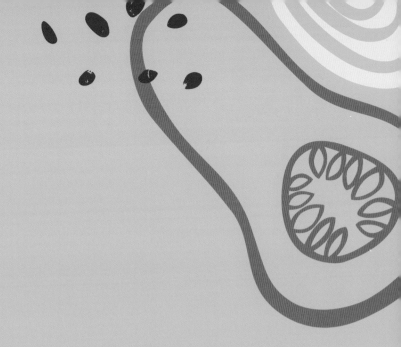

Classic Chicken Curry

Prep: **10 minutes**
(+ up to 24 hours marinating)

Cook: **50 minutes**

You know the kind of classic curry dish that everyone loves? This, my friends, is it. Chunks of chicken thighs are marinated in spiced yoghurt before being cooked in a tomato-based sauce for the perfect people-pleaser. It's miles better than a takeaway, and easy to make dairy-free too if coconut yoghurt is used. If you can find the time to marinate the chicken overnight, it will really elevate this dish to the next level.

600g chicken thighs, cut into large chunks

For the marinade
200g natural yoghurt or dairy-free alternative
2 tsp chopped garlic
2 tsp ginger paste
1 tsp salt
1 tsp ground turmeric
1 tsp garam masala
½ tsp ground black pepper

For the curry
1 tbsp vegetable oil
1 tsp cumin seeds
1 large onion, finely chopped
3 tsp chopped garlic
2 tsp ginger paste
1 x 400g tin chopped tomatoes
50g tomato purée
½ tsp salt
1 tsp ground turmeric
1 tsp garam masala
1 tsp chilli powder
2 tsp ground coriander
200ml water
2 tsp fenugreek leaves

Serves 4

1 Place the marinade ingredients in a large bowl and mix well. Add the chicken pieces, stirring to coat. Cover and leave in the fridge for at least 1 hour, or up to 24 hours if possible.

2 When you're ready to start cooking, heat the oil in a large pan over a medium heat. Add the cumin seeds and fry for 30 seconds, until they start to smell fragrant.

3 Add the onion and fry for 6–8 minutes, until the edges start to brown.

4 Add the garlic and ginger, stir well and fry for another minute.

5 Stir in the tomatoes and tomato purée and fry for another 2–3 minutes. Sprinkle in all the spices, apart from the fenugreek leaves, and mix well.

6 Add the marinated chicken to the pan along with the water. Stir to combine, then cover and bring the curry to the boil. Lower the heat to a simmer and cook for 30 minutes, stirring occasionally to ensure it doesn't stick.

7 When ready, sprinkle over the fenugreek leaves and stir. Cook for another 2–3 minutes, then turn off the heat, cover the pan and leave to rest for 5 minutes. If you want to freeze the curry, you can do so at this point. Allow to cool completely, then portion into tubs and pop in the freezer.

8 Serve with rice, samosas (see page 216), onion bhajis (see page 217), mango chutney and gluten-free naan breads (see page 209).

TOP TIP

Curries always taste better the next day, so if you can make this dish a day ahead and reheat it to serve, you're onto a winner.

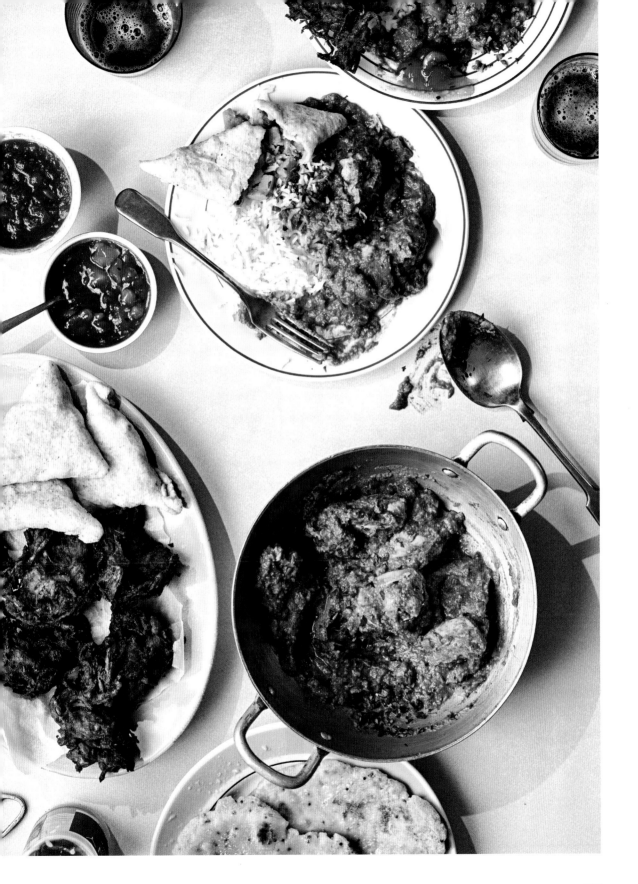

Sausage-Meat Pasta

Prep: **5 minutes**
Cook: **25 minutes**

EF **DF**

I remember my mum making this recipe all the time when I was a kid, and it went on to form the basis of my diet as a student. It was also one of the first recipes I ever published on my blog, and quickly became a firm favourite. Whatever weird and wonderful meals I conjure up in my imagination, you can bet I've always got a tub of this sauce stashed away in the freezer for a busy evening when I have no motivation to cook.

1 tbsp olive oil
6 gluten-free pork sausages, skin removed
1 small red onion, peeled and finely chopped
2 tsp chopped garlic
1 tsp dried basil
2 tsp dried oregano
1 tsp dried rosemary
1 x 400g tin chopped tomatoes
1 tbsp tomato purée
250g tomato passata
1 tsp balsamic vinegar
400g gluten-free pasta of choice
1 tbsp fresh basil leaves, chopped

Serves 4

1 Place the olive oil in a high-sided, non-stick pan over a medium-high heat. Once hot, add the skinned sausages and use a wooden spoon or spatula to break them up. Fry for 3–4 minutes, until the meat starts to brown and is in small chunks.

2 Add the onion and garlic and fry for another 2–3 minutes, stirring regularly.

3 Turn the heat down to medium, stir in the dried basil, oregano and rosemary and fry for another minute.

4 Add the tomatoes, tomato purée, passata and vinegar and stir well. Bring the sauce to the boil, then lower the heat and simmer for 10 minutes, stirring occasionally.

5 Meanwhile, cook the pasta in salted boiling water as per the packet instructions. When it is ready, reserve a tablespoon of the cooking water, then drain the pasta.

6 Add the fresh basil to the sauce and stir well. Any sauce that you won't be using straight away can be portioned into tubs, set aside until cold, then frozen.

7 Tip in the pasta into the pan of sauce along with the reserved cooking water and stir until the pasta is fully coated. Remove from the heat and serve straight away with a green salad.

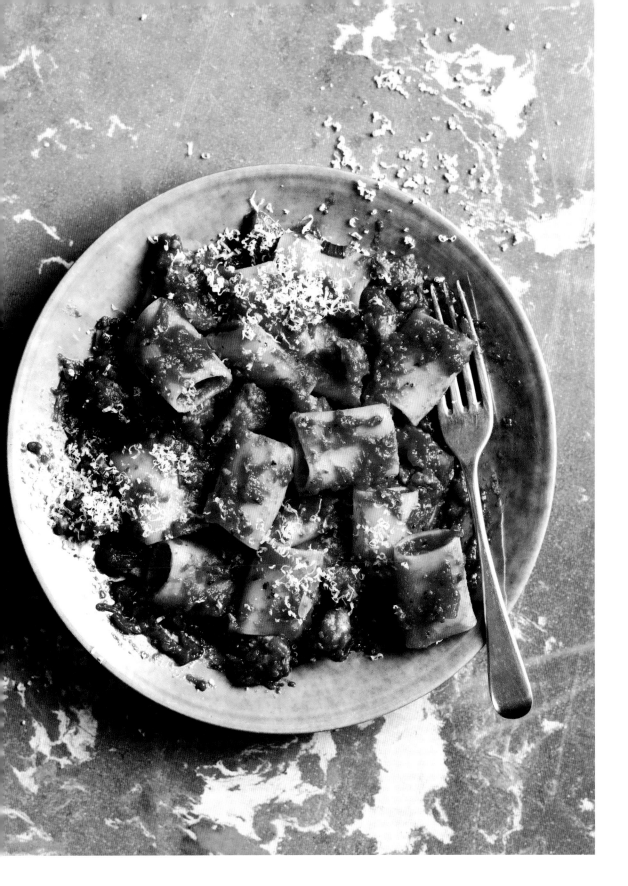

Spicy Turkey Burgers

Prep: **10 minutes**
Cook: **20 minutes**

I've always found homemade burgers a great meal to prepare in advance. You can freeze them cooked or uncooked, and cold leftovers can be chopped up and added to a salad or gluten-free wrap. These turkey burgers are packed with flavour and so easy to make that they're bound to become one of your midweek staples. I love to stack them high with homemade raita and mango chutney.

Vegetable oil, for greasing
500g lean turkey mince
1 onion, very finely chopped
50g gluten-free Panko Breadcrumbs (see page 38)
1 large egg
1 tsp dried coriander
1 tsp ground ginger
1 tsp ground cumin
1 tsp paprika
1 tsp cayenne pepper
1 tsp ground turmeric
½ tsp garlic granules
½ tsp salt

For the raita
¼ cucumber, grated
200g Greek yoghurt or dairy-free alternative
2 tbsp fresh coriander leaves, finely chopped
2 tbsp fresh mint leaves, finely chopped
Juice of ½ lemon
Pinch of salt

To serve
4 gluten-free burger buns
2 tbsp mango chutney
Lettuce

Serves 4

1 Preheat the oven to 200ºC/Fan 180ºC/Gas Mark 6 and lightly grease a roasting tray with a little oil.

2 Place the turkey mince in a large bowl, add the onion, breadcrumbs and egg and mix well.

3 Combine all the dried herbs, spices and salt in a small bowl, then sprinkle over the turkey mixture. Using your hands, 'squidge' the mixture together until it's completely combined, with no loose spices or breadcrumbs visible.

4 Divide the mixture into 8 equal pieces – you can weigh them for accuracy – and roll each one into a ball. Use your hands to flatten the balls into patties about 2cm thick, then place them spaced apart on the roasting tray. If you like, you can freeze the burgers at this stage between sheets of baking paper so they don't stick together.

5 Roast the burgers for 20 minutes, turning halfway through, until browned and well cooked.

6 Meanwhile, make the raita. Squeeze any excess moisture out of the cucumber, then add to a bowl with the other raita ingredients and mix well.

7 When the burgers are cooked, serve in the buns, topping each burger with a dollop of raita, some mango chutney and lettuce. Any cooked burgers that are left over can be frozen once they have cooled completely.

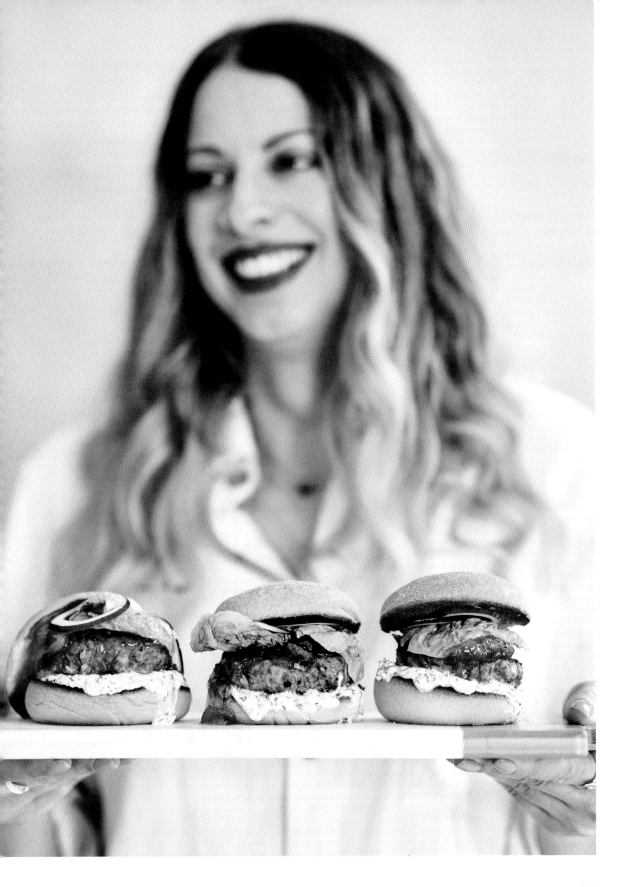

Meatball Chilli Con Carne

Prep: **15 minutes**
Cook: **35 minutes**

DF

I love meatballs, and I adore chilli con carne, so since I had an early hours epiphany about combining the two, I've honestly never looked back. The best thing about this recipe is that you can either batch-cook and freeze portions of the entire dish, or just make and freeze extra meatballs for an easier job next time you cook this. Either way, it's fantastic served with rice and topped with sour cream and cheese.

500g beef mince, at least 10% fat
1 large egg
40g gluten-free Panko Breadcrumbs (see page 38)
1 tsp garlic granules
1 tsp onion salt
1 tsp chilli powder
1 tsp ground cumin
1 tbsp olive oil

For the chilli bean sauce
1 large onion, finely chopped
2 tsp chopped garlic
1 tsp chilli powder

1 tsp paprika
1 tsp ground cumin
1 x 400g tin chopped tomatoes
200ml tomato passata
1 tsp dried marjoram
1 gluten-free beef stock pot
1 x 400g tin kidney beans, drained
1 square of dark chocolate (about 10g), at least 70% cocoa solids

To serve
120g Cheddar cheese, grated
100ml soured cream

Serves 4

1   To make the meatballs, place the beef in a large bowl and add the egg, breadcrumbs and flavourings. Use your hands to 'squish' the mixture together for at least a minute, until it is completely combined.

2   Divide the mixture into 20 equal pieces weighing about 30g each. Roll them into balls.

3   Place the oil in a large frying pan over a high heat. When hot, fry the meatballs in batches for 4–5 minutes, turning often until they are brown on all sides. Transfer to a plate.

4   To make the chilli and bean sauce, return the oily pan to a medium-low heat and fry the onion for 4–5 minutes, until translucent and golden around the edges.

5   Add the garlic, chilli powder, paprika and cumin to the pan, mix well and fry for another 2 minutes.

6   Add the tomatoes, passata, marjoram and stock pot to the pan and mix well. Return the meatballs and any of their juices to the pan. Stir well, then lower the heat, cover with a lid and simmer for 10 minutes, stirring once or twice to prevent sticking.

7   After 10 minutes, add the kidney beans and chocolate to the pan. Mix well, cover again and simmer for another 10 minutes. At this point the dish can be set aside to cool before freezing.

8   Serve the meatball chilli with rice, topped with the grated cheese and soured cream.

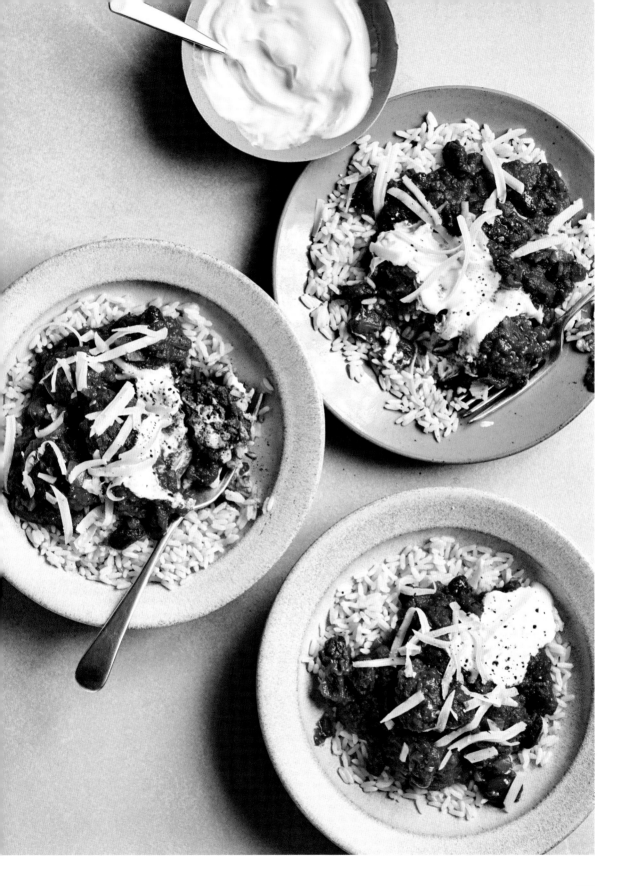

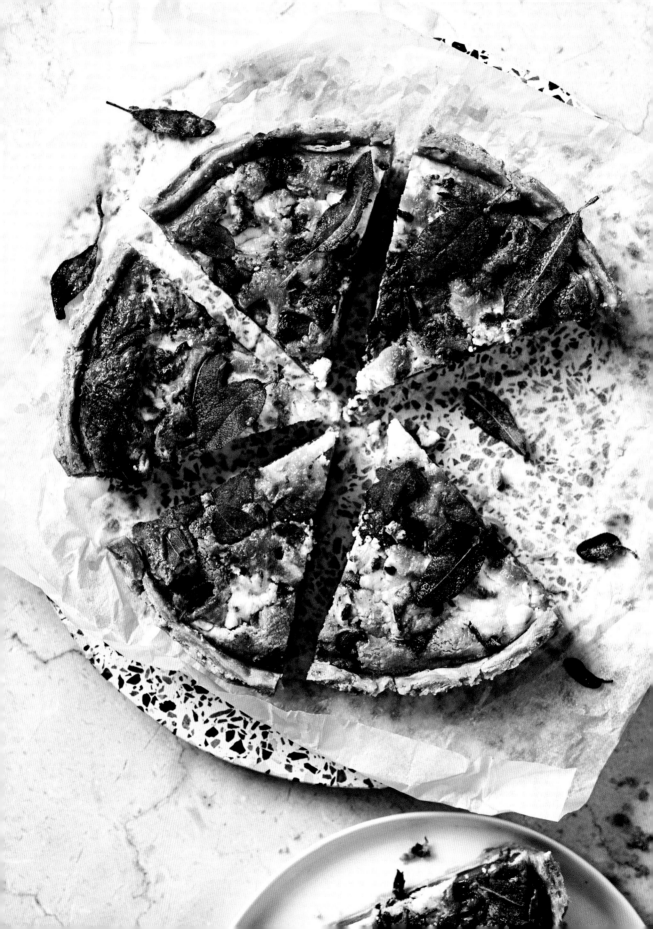

Butternut Squash & Goats' Cheese Quiche

20g salted butter
Small handful of fresh sage
  (about 15 leaves)
500g frozen butternut squash
  chunks
1 tbsp olive oil
1 tsp dried chilli flakes

Gluten-free plain flour, for
  dusting
½ quantity chilled Shortcrust
  Pastry (see page 39)
3 large eggs
150ml double cream
75g soft goats' cheese
Salt and pepper

Prep: **15 minutes**
Cook: **1¼ hours**

There's something about the combination of creamy goats' cheese, sweet butternut squash and crispy sage that makes a particularly dreamy quiche. Enjoy it hot or cold as part of a picnic, as a scrumptious sandwich alternative for lunchboxes, or as a lovely light meal for summer evenings.

Serves 6-8

1   Preheat the oven to 200ºC/Fan 180ºC/Gas Mark 6. Set out a 23cm quiche dish.

2   Place the butter in a small frying pan over a medium heat. Once melted, add the sage leaves and fry for 1–2 minutes, until crispy. Remove with tongs and set to one side.

3   Place the squash in a large roasting tray. Pour in the melted butter from the frying pan, then add the olive oil, chilli flakes and a pinch of salt. Toss to coat the squash, then roast for 30 minutes, turning the chunks halfway through. Remove from the oven and lower the heat to 180ºC/Fan 160ºC/Gas Mark 4.

4   Flour a work surface and place the chilled pastry on it. Roll it out to a thickness of about 4mm, then use it to line your quiche dish. Trim off the excess, then blind-bake it as described on page 39.

5   Meanwhile, place the eggs and cream in a large bowl, ideally one with a pouring lip, and whisk briefly to combine. Add the roasted squash and crispy sage leaves, then crumble in the goats' cheese and stir well.

6   Remove the pastry case from the oven and carefully pour in the egg mixture, taking care that it does not overflow. Make sure the squash and goats' cheese are evenly distributed, then return the case to the oven for another 35–40 minutes, until the quiche is golden on top and does not wobble in the centre.

7   Serve hot or cold with a green salad, or even some gluten-free oven chips if you're feeling cheeky.

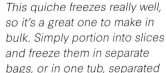

TOP TIP

This quiche freezes really well, so it's a great one to make in bulk. Simply portion into slices and freeze them in separate bags, or in one tub, separated by baking paper.

Ultimate Mac & Cheese

400g gluten-free macaroni
50g unsalted butter, plus an extra knob
2 tsp chopped garlic
50g gluten-free plain flour
500ml milk
275g mature Cheddar cheese, grated

75g mozzarella cheese, grated
4 processed cheese slices

For the topping
45g gluten-free breadcrumbs
50g Cheddar cheese, grated

Prep: **5 minutes**
Cook: **30 minutes**

 MF   EF

I remember eating the most incredible gluten-free mac and cheese in New York City, and this recipe is the result of about ten years of trying to recreate that exact meal. This really is my favourite comfort food, and baking it with a cheesy crumb topping is the pièce de résistance. If you want to make portions to freeze, I recommend following the recipe up to step 6, then dividing it between foil trays and adding the topping. Simply cover and freeze until needed. The portions can be reheated from frozen in 30 minutes at 200ºC/Fan 180ºC/Gas Mark 6 – just like a ready meal, but miles better.

Serves 4

1   Preheat the oven to 200ºC/Fan 180ºC/Gas Mark 6.

2   Bring a pan of salted water to the boil and cook the macaroni in it for 5–6 minutes, until al dente.

3   While the water is heating and the pasta is cooking, place the butter and garlic in a large saucepan over a low heat. Once the butter has melted, gently fry the garlic for a further 2 minutes.

4   Add the flour and use a whisk to mix into a thick paste. Continue to cook for 30–60 seconds, stirring constantly so it doesn't stick.

5   Pour in about 100ml of the milk and stir constantly until it forms a smooth, thick paste. Continue adding the milk about 100ml at a time, stirring constantly after each addition, until the mixture is smooth again. Once all the milk has been added, you should have a smooth, thick white sauce.

6   Drain the macaroni, then pour back into its pan and stir in a knob of butter until melted. Set to one side.

7   Add the grated Cheddar and mozzarella to the white sauce, then crumble in the cheese slices. Stir until all the cheese has melted, then remove from the heat.

8   Add the cooked macaroni to the sauce and mix well. Pour the mixture into a 23cm ovenproof dish, then sprinkle with the breadcrumb and cheese toppings. Bake for 20 minutes, until the surface is golden and bubbling.

9   Serve with a good helping of peas or a fresh green salad.

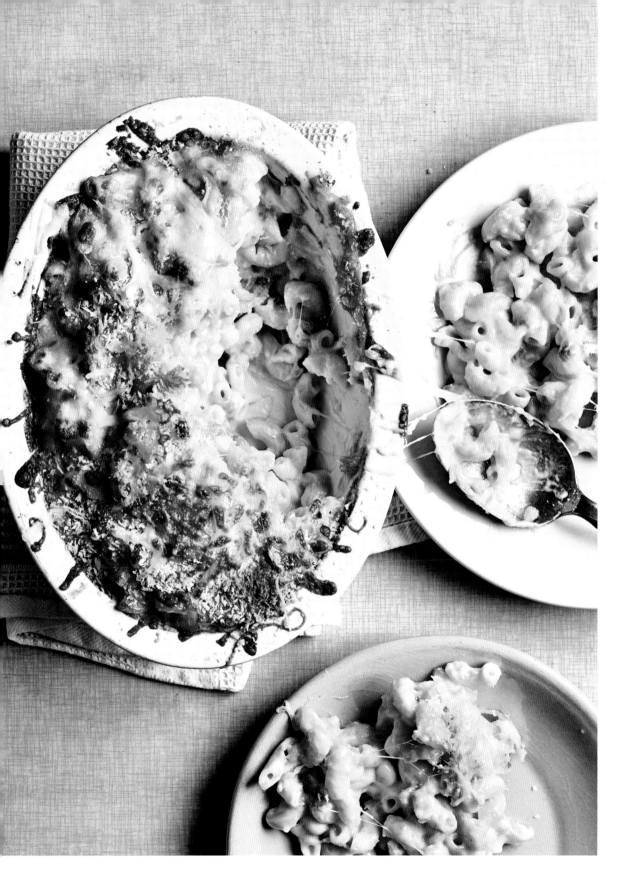

Chicken, Ham & Leek Puff Pie

30g unsalted butter
1 celery stick, finely chopped
1 onion, finely chopped
2 carrots, finely chopped
1 leek, finely sliced
30g gluten-free plain flour
400ml milk

1 gluten-free vegetable
  stock pot
1 tsp dried tarragon
200g chopped cooked ham
200g shredded cooked chicken
1 quantity chilled Rough
  Puff Pastry (see page 40)
1 egg, beaten

Prep: **15 minutes**
Cook: **1 hour**

Some might argue that a pie with no walls isn't truly a pie. But when it tastes this good, who cares? This is my go-to recipe for using up roast dinner leftovers, and at Christmas I switch the chicken for turkey and make a Boxing Day version. If you like, you can batch-cook the filling in advance, then simply bake with the puff pastry lid when you fancy it. The tarragon goes really well with chicken, making this comfort food at its finest.

Serves 4

1   Melt the butter in a large saucepan over a low heat, then add the celery, onion, carrots and leek. Fry gently for 6–8 minutes until the vegetables have softened.

2   Stir the flour into the pan, mix well and cook for 30 seconds.

3   Pour in the milk about a third at a time, mixing well between each addition to ensure there are no lumps. Once you have a smooth sauce, add the stock and the tarragon. Stir well over a low heat, until the stock has dissolved and you have a thick, white sauce.

4   Turn off the heat, stir in the ham and chicken, then leave to cool for about 30 minutes.

5   Once the pie mixture has cooled, preheat the oven to 200°C/Fan 180°C/Gas Mark 6. Transfer the filling to a 23cm pie dish and spread evenly.

6   Place the chilled pastry between 2 sheets of clingfilm and roll it out to a thickness of 4mm. Don't knead or reroll the pastry at all or you'll lose the lovely layers. Place a plate the same diameter as your pie dish on the pastry and cut around it. Brush the rim of the dish with water, then carefully place the pastry over the whole dish. Cut a steam hole in the centre, then brush the top with the beaten egg. If you like, stamp small decorative shapes from the offcuts, without rerolling the pastry, and stick them to the top of the pie, before brushing again with beaten egg.

7   Bake the pie for 20 minutes, until the pastry is golden.

8   Serve with green veg and a helping of mashed potato or gluten-free oven chips.

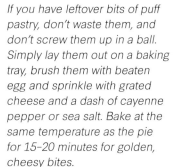

TOP TIP ▶▶▶▶▶

If you have leftover bits of puff pastry, don't waste them, and don't screw them up in a ball. Simply lay them out on a baking tray, brush them with beaten egg and sprinkle with grated cheese and a dash of cayenne pepper or sea salt. Bake at the same temperature as the pie for 15–20 minutes for golden, cheesy bites.

98

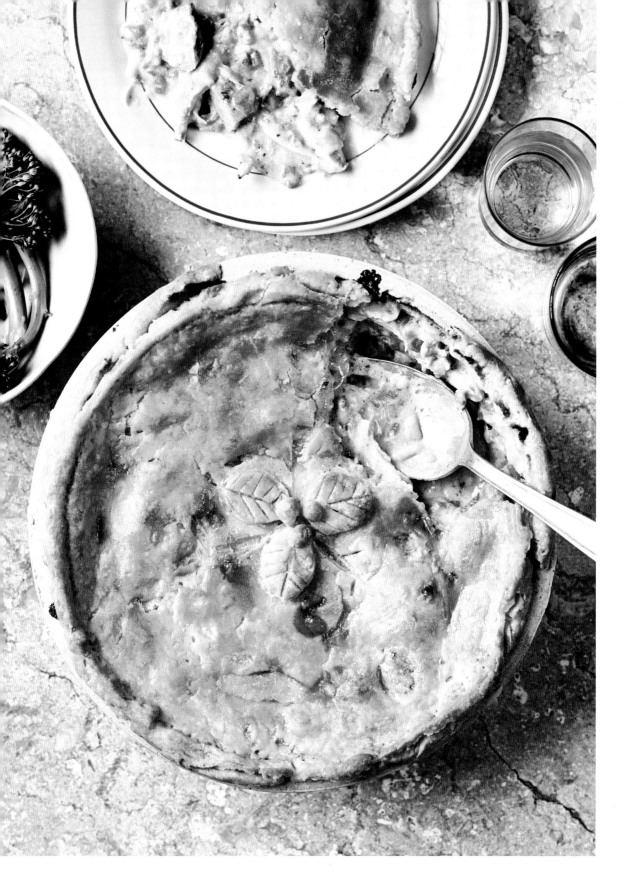

Fantastic Fish Pie

Prep: **15 minutes**
Cook: **45 minutes**

450ml milk
1 bay leaf
400g mixture of skinless cod,
  smoked haddock and salmon,
  chopped into chunks
50g unsalted butter
1 onion, finely chopped
1 tsp chopped garlic
50g gluten-free plain flour
1 tbsp Dijon mustard
1 tbsp tomato ketchup

170g raw king prawns, shelled
100g frozen peas
Salt and pepper

For the topping
1kg Maris Piper potatoes,
  peeled and cut into 5cm
  chunks
35g unsalted butter
200g mature Cheddar cheese,
  grated

I love a good fish pie, an oozing, golden mess of yumminess. In fact, the messier the sauce and cheese dripping down the side of the dish, the better in my opinion. It's a pub classic, but a gluten-free version is really hard to find. That's where this recipe comes in. It's packed with white fish, smoked fish, salmon and prawns in a creamy sauce and topped with the cheesiest mash in the world – a plate of pure comfort.

Serves 4

1 Preheat the oven to 200ºC/Fan 180ºC/Gas Mark 6. Bring a large pan of salted water to the boil, add the potato chunks and boil for 15 minutes, until a knife slips in easily. Drain, return to the pan and set aside.

2 Meanwhile, place the milk and bay leaf in a pan and heat until hot but not boiling – you don't want it bubbling. Add the fish chunks and keep on a low heat for 4–5 minutes, being careful not to let it boil. Using a slotted spoon, transfer the fish to a plate and set aside. Discard the bay leaf but keep the milk in the pan.

3 Place the butter in a separate pan and melt over a low–medium heat. Add the onion and garlic and fry gently for 3–4 minutes, until translucent.

4 Stir in the flour and use a balloon whisk to combine the mixture into a thick paste. Continue to cook for 30–60 seconds, stirring constantly so it doesn't stick.

5 Pour in about 100ml of the reserved milk and keep stirring until it forms a smooth, thick paste. Continue adding the milk about 100ml at a time, stirring constantly until all the lumps are gone. Once you have a smooth, thick sauce, stir in the mustard and ketchup, generously season with salt and pepper, then take off the heat.

6 Add the fish, prawns and peas to the sauce, stirring gently until well combined. You want to avoid breaking up the fish too much. Pour the mixture into a 23cm round ovenproof dish.

7 To make the topping, add the butter and three-quarters of the cheese to the drained potatoes and mash until smooth. Spoon the mixture evenly over the saucy fish mixture in the

TOP TIP

Planning to freeze this pie for future use? Divide the fish mixture equally between foil trays, then top with the mash and a sprinkling of cheese. Freeze once cooled. When needed, simply defrost and reheat at 200ºC/Fan 180ºC/Gas Mark 6 for 30 minutes. Make sure it is hot throughout before serving.

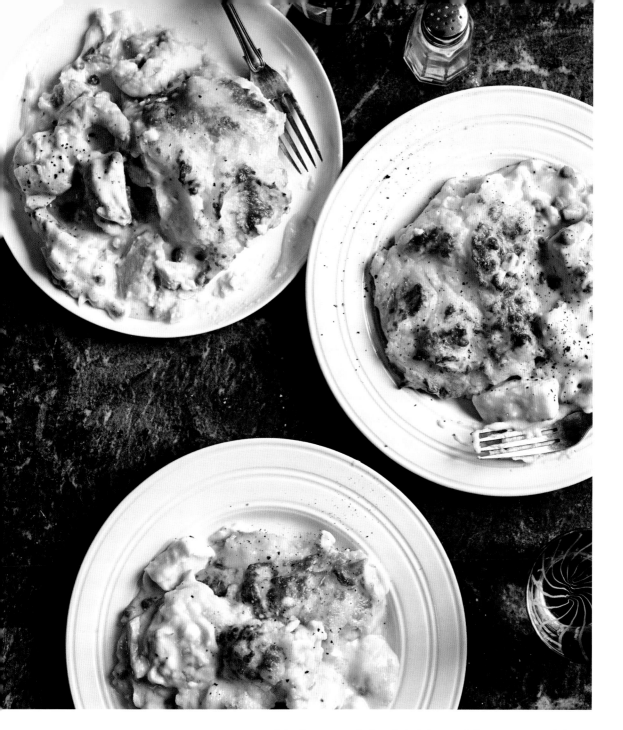

dish, then use a fork to 'rake' the mash into one smooth layer. Top with the remaining cheese.

8 Place the dish in a roasting tray to catch any 'over-excited' sauce, then bake for 30 minutes, until the cheesy mash is golden and the sauce is bubbling up.

9 Serve with a good helping of peas and sweetcorn.

Banging Bolognese

Prep: **10 minutes**
Cook: **1 hour**

2 tbsp virgin olive oil, plus a little extra for the pasta
2 onions, peeled and finely chopped
2 celery sticks, finely chopped
1 carrot, finely chopped
3 garlic cloves, peeled and crushed
2 tbsp dried basil
1 tbsp dried oregano

500g beef mince, at least 10% fat
1 x 400g tin chopped tomatoes
300ml tomato passata
125ml red wine
2 tbsp tomato purée
1 gluten-free beef stock pot
400g gluten-free spaghetti
1 tbsp fresh basil leaves
2 tbsp grated Parmesan cheese or dairy-free alternative

It's a fact of life that my dad makes the best spag bol around, but he refuses to divulge his recipe, even though I've spent years trying to wheedle it out of him. Happily, my version comes a very close second. To me, making bolognese is a true joy, and a perfect example of how good things take time. It's even better if you make it the day before and leave the flavours to develop in the fridge overnight. Also, any leftovers make a great pizza topping in place of a classic tomato sauce.

Serves 4

1 Place half the olive oil in a large, non-stick pan over a low heat. When hot, add the onions, celery, carrot and garlic and fry for 5–7 minutes, stirring occasionally, until everything begins to soften and the onions are translucent.

2 Add the remaining oil to the pan, along with the dried basil and oregano. Stir to mix, then increase the heat to medium-high. Once the pan is sizzling, add the beef and use a wooden spoon or silicone spatula to break it up. Keep stirring and chopping until it is all brown and there are no pink bits left, about another 4–5 minutes.

3 Add the tomatoes, passata, red wine, tomato purée and stock pot to the pan. Mix well and bring to the boil. When bubbling, turn the heat right down, cover with a lid and leave to simmer for 45 minutes. Stir occasionally to ensure it's not sticking. If you want to freeze any of the finished sauce, portion it into tubs and allow to cool completely before popping in the freezer.

4 About 15–20 minutes before the sauce has finished cooking, bring a pan of salted water to the boil. Add a drop of olive oil, then cook the spaghetti as per the packet instructions. When it's ready, reserve 2 tablespoons of the cooking water, then drain the spaghetti.

5 Once the bolognese sauce is ready, add the spaghetti plus the reserved pasta water and stir well, using a pasta spoon or tongs.

6 Serve sprinkled with torn fresh basil leaves and grated Parmesan.

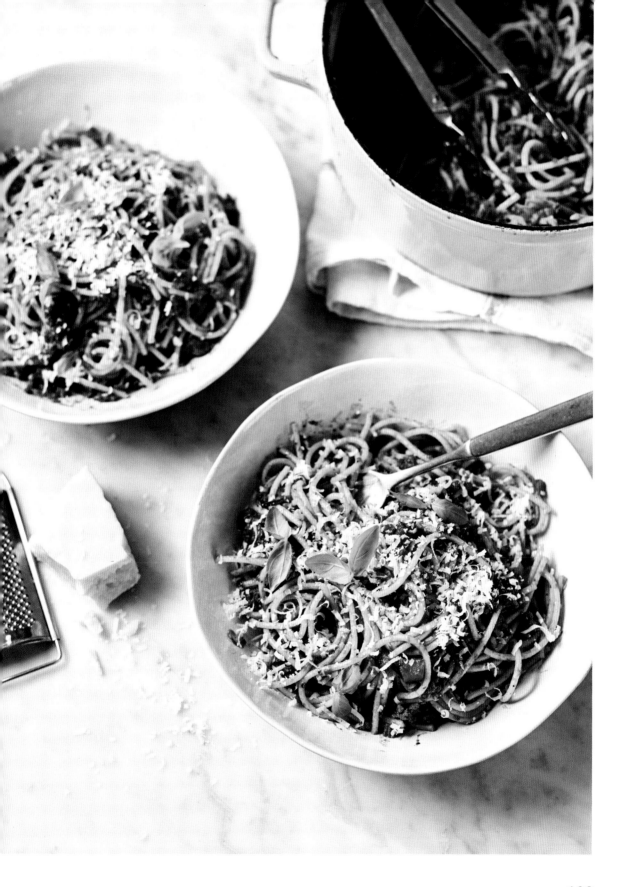

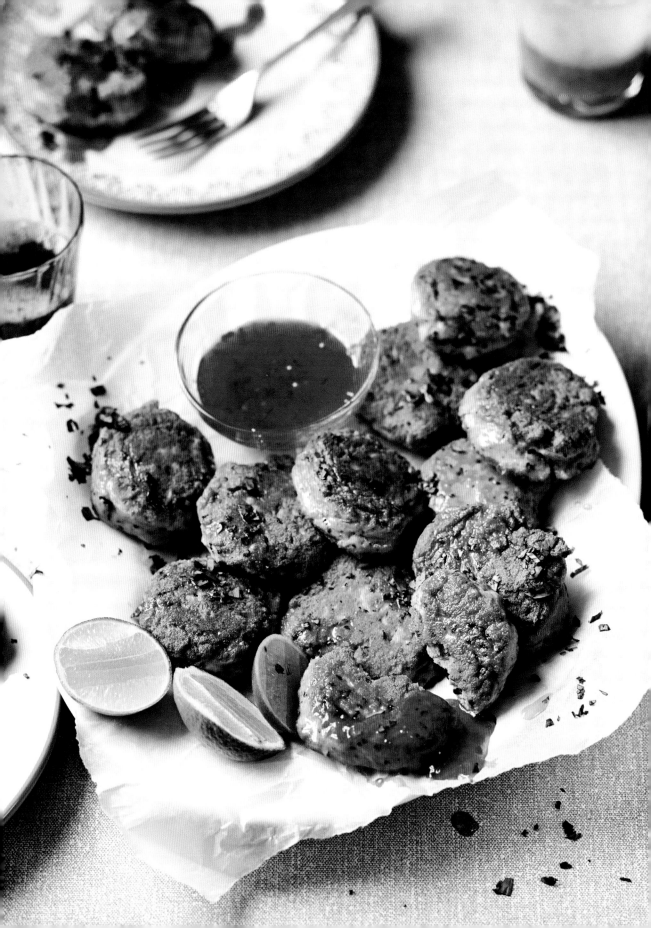

Thai Salmon Fishcakes

600g skinless and boneless
  salmon fillets
2 tbsp Thai red curry paste
Zest of 2 limes
Handful of coriander

4 spring onions, chopped
2 eggs
2 tbsp gluten-free plain flour
2 tbsp vegetable oil
Sweet chilli sauce, to serve

Prep: **10 minutes**
Cook: **10 minutes**

DF

These fishcakes are great as part of a buffet-style meal and just as tasty for a light lunch, served with a crunchy salad. If making a big batch, you can either freeze the uncooked patties on a baking tray, then pop them in a bag once frozen so they don't lose their shape, or freeze them once cooked and heat before eating.

Serves 4

1 Place all the ingredients, except the oil and chilli sauce, in a food processor and blitz until it forms a mousse-like consistency.

2 Divide the mixture into 16 equal pieces – about 1 heaped tablespoon each – and use wet hands to shape them into patties 2–3cm thick.

3 Heat the oil in a large frying pan. When hot, add half the patties. Fry for 2 minutes on each side, until brown. Transfer to a plate and fry the remaining patties.

4 Serve the fishcakes hot with a mixed salad and sweet chilli sauce for dipping. You can also cut the zested lime into wedges to squeeze on the fishcakes before eating.

Chickpea & Potato Curry

1 tbsp vegetable oil
1 large onion, finely chopped
4 tsp chopped garlic
2 tsp ginger paste
1 tsp salt
1 tsp ground turmeric
1 tsp chilli powder
2 tsp garam masala

1 x 400g tin chickpeas in water, drained
500g baby potatoes
1 x 400g tin chopped tomatoes
1 tbsp tomato purée
200ml full-fat coconut milk
1 tbsp mango chutney
200g frozen chopped spinach
Handful of fresh coriander

Prep: **5 minutes**
Cook: **40 minutes**

 EF **DF** **V**

Here is a multitasking dish that is both an excellent meat-free meal and a great side dish for any curry feast. It can be made conventionally, or in a slow cooker. In fact, I originally posted this recipe on my Instagram channel as a slow cooker staple and it quickly went viral. Check out the tips below if you want to slow-cook it yourself. Also note that it freezes well.

Serves 4

1   Place the oil in a large pan over a medium heat. Once hot, add the onion and fry for 6–8 minutes, until golden.

2   Add the garlic and ginger and fry for another minute. Add the salt, turmeric, chilli powder and garam masala, mix well and fry for another 30 seconds.

3   Now add the chickpeas and potatoes to the pan and mix well to coat them in the spices.

4   Add the tomatoes, tomato purée, coconut milk, mango chutney and frozen spinach and stir well. Bring to the boil, then lower the heat to a simmer and cover the pan with a lid. Cook for 30 minutes, stirring occasionally. When the time is up, remove the lid and cook for a further 5 minutes.

5   Sprinkle the finished dish with the coriander and serve. Any leftovers can be portioned into tubs and cooled completely before freezing.

 SLOW COOKER SWAP

Place everything apart from the spinach and coriander in your slow cooker and cook on high for 3–4 hours, or low for 5–6 hours. In the last 30 minutes, add the frozen spinach and mix well. Replace the lid and leave to finish cooking. Serve with the coriander sprinkled on top.

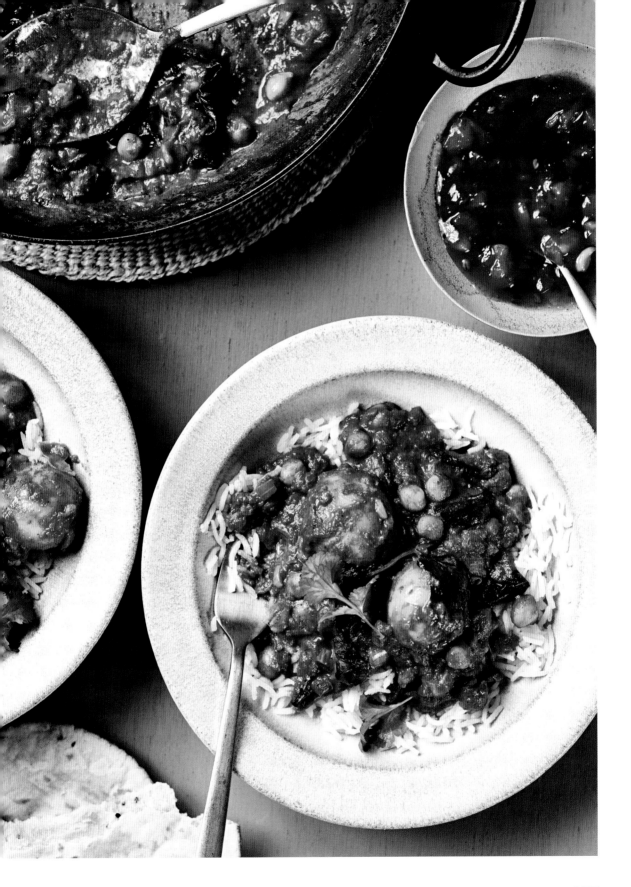

Stuffed Cannelloni

Prep: **45 minutes**
Cook: **1¼ hours**

I have fond memories of my pre-coeliac days, when I ate cannelloni tubes stuffed with gorgeous bites of spinach and stringy mozzarella slathered in a rich and garlicky tomato sauce. Those memories led me to try recreating that experience using homemade, gluten-free pasta. It's actually surprisingly simple, and you don't even need a pasta maker. Once you try it, I'm sure you'll be converted.

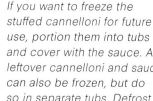

TOP TIP

If you want to freeze the stuffed cannelloni for future use, portion them into tubs and cover with the sauce. Any leftover cannelloni and sauce can also be frozen, but do so in separate tubs. Defrost completely, then cook as above – or add an extra 15 minutes to cook straight from frozen.

1 quantity Fresh Pasta dough
  (see page 36)
Gluten-free flour, for dusting
150g Cheddar cheese, grated
20g Parmesan cheese, grated

For the filling
15g butter
150g baby spinach leaves
250g ricotta cheese
30g Parmesan cheese, grated
125g mozzarella cheese, cut into
  small pieces

Salt and pepper

For the sauce
1 tbsp olive oil
1 onion, finely chopped
2 tsp chopped garlic
2 tsp dried oregano
1 tsp dried basil
1 tsp chilli flakes
2 x 400g tins finely chopped
  tomatoes
2 tbsp tomato purée

Serves 4

1 Start by making the sauce. Place the olive oil in a pan over a medium heat. Once hot, add the onion and garlic and fry for 6–8 minutes, until soft.

2 Sprinkle in the oregano, basil and chilli flakes, then stir-fry for a further 30 seconds.

3 Add the tomatoes and tomato purée, mix well and bring to the boil. Lower the heat to a simmer and leave for 5 minutes, stirring occasionally. Set to one side.

4 Divide the pasta dough into 4 equal pieces and wrap 3 of them in clingfilm so they don't dry out. Generously dust a sheet of baking paper with the flour, then place the unwrapped piece of dough on it. Roll into a rectangle about 30 x 12cm and 1–2mm thick – it should be thin enough to see through. Keep turning the pasta to ensure it doesn't stick, and add extra flour if needed. It should be smooth and not at all sticky.

5 Trim the edges of the pasta to straighten them, then cut the rectangle widthways into 3 equal pieces measuring 10 x 12cm. Use a pastry brush to dust off as much flour as possible, then place the rectangles on a clean sheet of baking paper. Repeat this step with each piece of pasta dough until you have 12 rectangles in total. Leave these all on the clean baking paper to dry slightly while you make the filling.

6 Melt the butter in a frying pan over a medium heat. Add the spinach and fry for 1–2 minutes, until wilted. Transfer to a large bowl, add all the remaining filling ingredients and mix well with a fork.

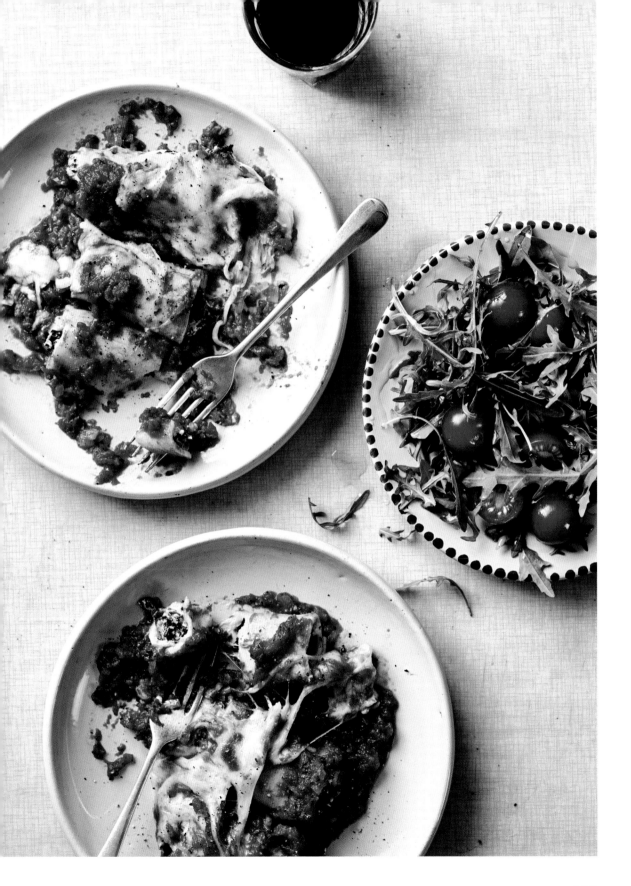

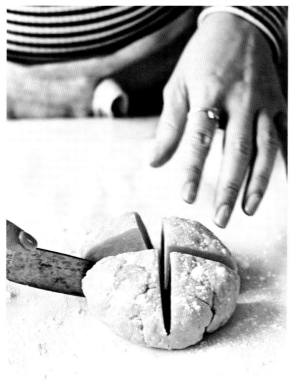

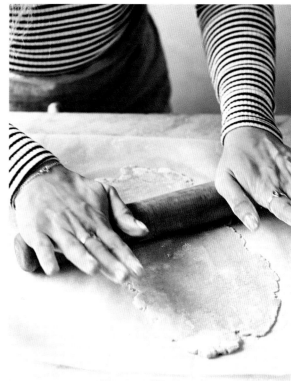

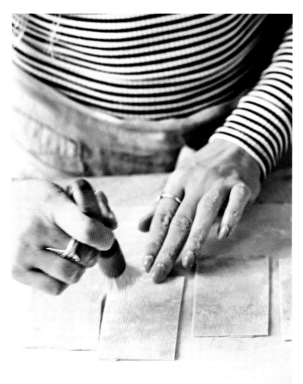

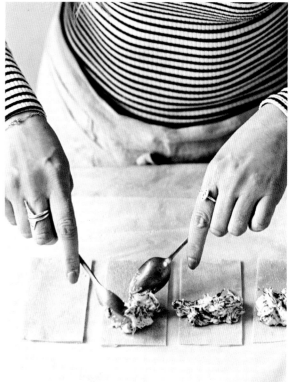

110

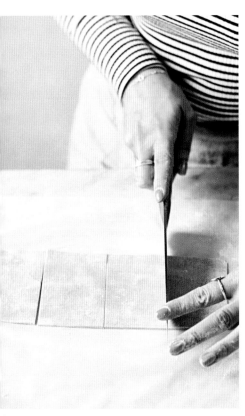

7 Preheat the oven to 200°C/Fan 180°C/Gas Mark 6.

8 Place about 1 heaped tablespoon of the filling at the short end of a pasta sheet, arrange in a sausage shape across the width, then roll up to form a tube. Repeat with each rectangle of pasta. To ensure the filling is distributed equally, you can either weigh it and divide that weight by 12, or distribute the filling as equally as you can between all 12 sheets before rolling them up.

9 Take a heaped spoonful or so of the tomato sauce and slather it in an even layer in the bottom of a baking dish that is large enough to hold all the cannelloni in one layer. This will ensure the pasta cooks evenly and doesn't stick.

10 Place the cannelloni in the dish – it doesn't matter if they're touching – and pour the remaining sauce over them. They should be completely covered. Sprinkle with the grated cheeses and bake for 45–50 minutes, until the top is golden and the sauce is bubbling. Serve with a crunchy green salad.

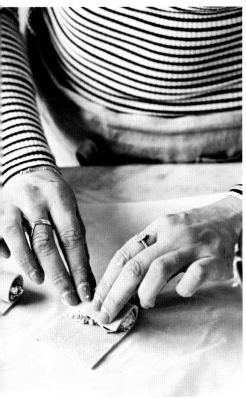

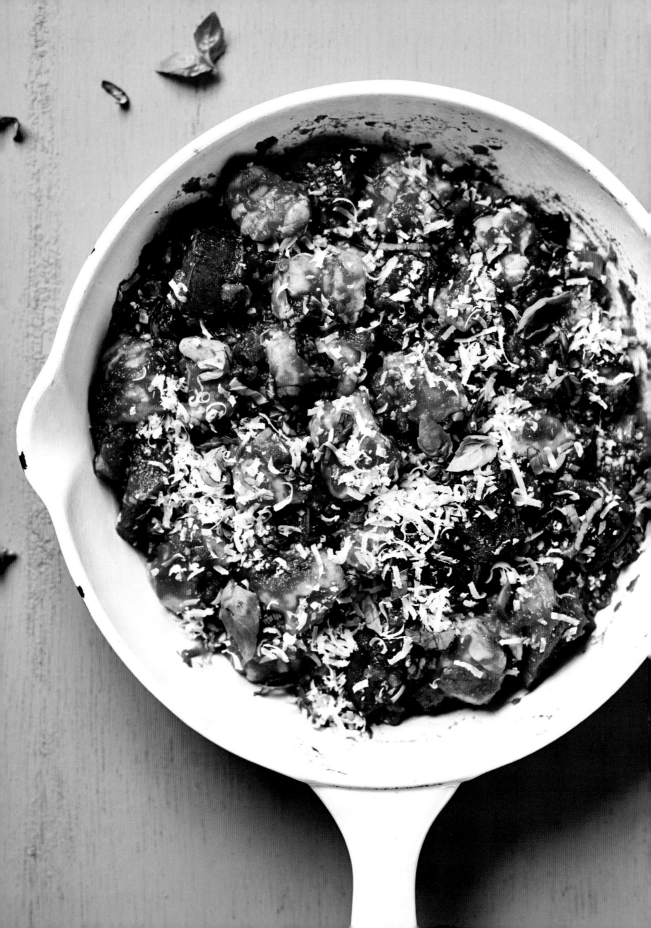

ONE-PAN WONDERS

I do love a good one-pan meal, not least because I absolutely hate washing up. It saves time standing at the sink and can save on your energy bills too. The methods below also give cooking options, depending on whether you want to hang around in the kitchen stirring something on the hob, or shove a meal in the oven while you get on with something more interesting.

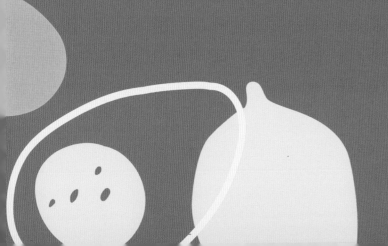

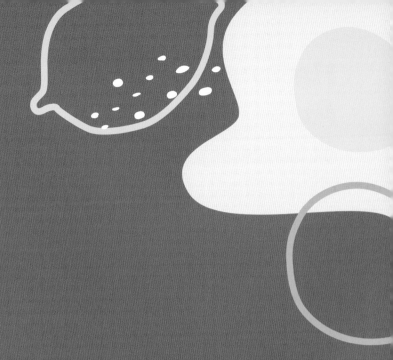

THE RECIPES

Halloumi, Aubergine & Chickpea Traybake

1 aubergine
1 large sweet potato
  (about 500g)
1 red pepper
1 x 400g tin chickpeas, drained
1 tbsp olive oil
45g harissa paste
225g halloumi cheese

For the garlic yoghurt
2 tbsp natural fat-free yoghurt
1 tsp chopped garlic
1 tsp olive oil
Salt and pepper
Chopped fresh parsley

Prep: **5 minutes**
Cook: **45 minutes**

I like to think of this as a dish for 'reluctant vegetarians' – those who are trying to cut down their meat consumption even though they love it. The aubergine, halloumi and chickpeas add lots of texture, so are great replacements for meat, and really filling at the same time. Pairing the spicy harissa dressing with a creamy yoghurt drizzle provides extra wow.

Serves 4

1   Preheat the oven to 200ºC/Fan 180ºC/Gas Mark 6. Set out a non-stick roasting tray.

2   Slice the aubergine and sweet potato into rounds about 1cm thick, then cut each round into quarters. Place in a large bowl.

3   Deseed the red pepper, cut into large chunks and add to the bowl along with the chickpeas. Drizzle with the olive oil and add the harissa pasta. Mix well so everything is coated, then tip the mixture into your roasting tray. Spread out evenly, then place in the oven for 30 minutes.

4   Slice the halloumi into 8 pieces, lay them over the vegetable mixture and return the tray to the oven for another 10–15 minutes, until the veg has cooked through.

5   Meanwhile, place the yoghurt, garlic and olive oil in a small bowl, add salt and pepper and mix together. Drizzle this mixture over the veg tray, then sprinkle with chopped parsley. Serve straight away.

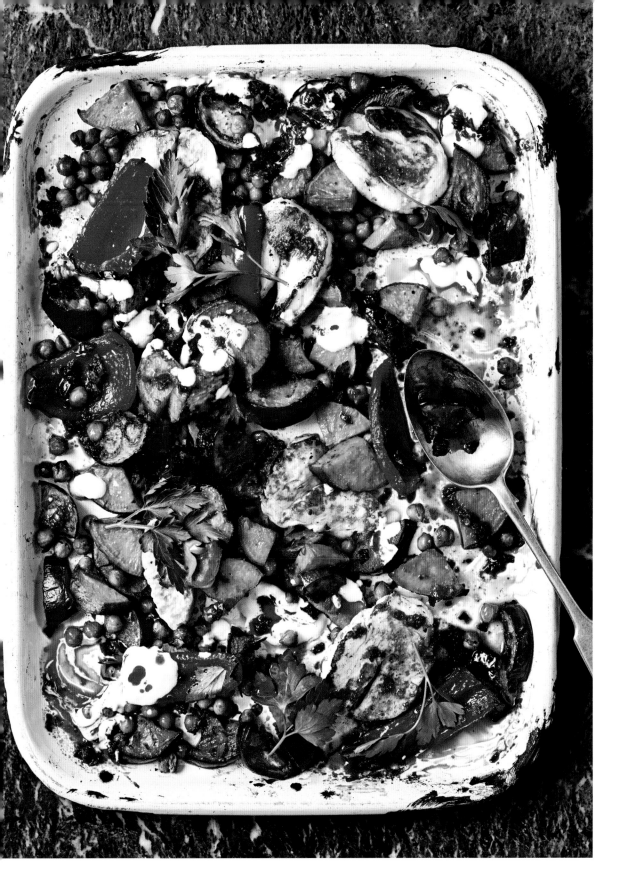

Bacon & Brie Gnocchi Bake

1 tbsp olive oil
260g smoked bacon lardons
1 onion, finely chopped
1 tsp chopped garlic
1 tsp dried thyme
150ml mild gluten-free vegetable
    stock (see Tip below)

260g baby spinach
250g full-fat cream cheese
200g Brie cheese, cut into slices
    2.5cm long
1 quantity gluten-free gnocchi
    (see page 34)

Prep: **5 minutes**
Cook: **30 minutes**

There's something about the combination of bacon and Brie that just screams comfort food – and when you add in pillowy gnocchi and a creamy garlic sauce, you've peaked. This is a dish for when you're craving something indulgent, though the addition of gorgeously green spinach means you can at least pretend it's a little healthy.

Serves 4

1 Preheat the oven to 200ºC/Fan 180ºC/Gas Mark 6.

2 Place the oil in a large ovenproof pan over a medium heat. Once hot, add the bacon lardons and fry for 5 minutes, until they start to brown and crisp up.

3 Add the onion, garlic and dried thyme, and continue to fry for another 3–4 minutes.

4 Pour in the stock and use a spatula to stir and scrape up any bits stuck to the bottom of the pan. Add the spinach and stir over a low heat for a minute or so, until it has wilted.

5   Add the cream cheese and stir until it has combined with the liquid to form a smooth sauce. Add half the Brie and the uncooked gnocchi and stir well so the gnocchi is completely coated in the sauce and the Brie is evenly distributed throughout.

6 Top the gnocchi with the remaining pieces of Brie, then place the pan in the oven for 15 minutes, until the Brie is bubbling. If you like, you can grill it for the final couple of minutes to get a lovely, browned effect on the topping.

TOP TIP

As the bacon is salty, and stock is too, I always make a mild stock for this recipe, dissolving 1 gluten-free stock cube in 800ml boiling water, before measuring out what I need. Any leftover stock can be kept for future recipes, or used for cooking some veg that can then be blended to make soup.

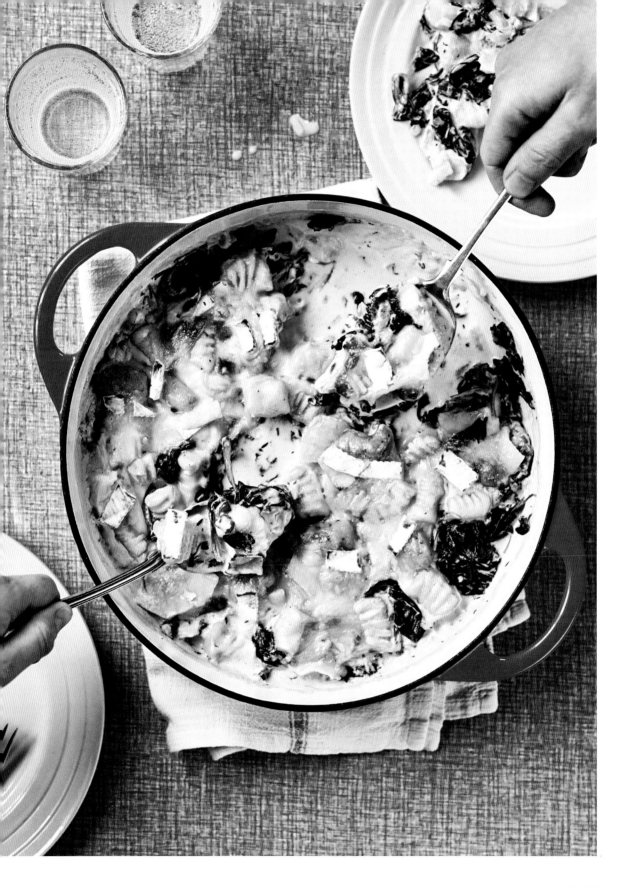

Creamy Vegetable Pot Pie

Prep: **10 minutes**
Cook: **45 minutes**

For those evenings when you want the joy of a pie without any faff, this is the perfect recipe. All you need to do is whip up the creamy vegetable stew, pop the pastry lid on top and chuck the whole thing in the oven for a pretty effortless meal. What's more, it's packed full of vegetables and creamy butter beans, making it a vegetarian meal that even the meat-eaters of the house will love.

50g unsalted butter
2 leeks, sliced
1 celery stick, finely chopped
1 red onion, finely chopped
250g carrots, chopped into 1cm chunks
200g baby chestnut mushrooms, or bigger ones cut in half
75g frozen peas
75g frozen sweetcorn
1 tsp dried rosemary
1 tsp dried thyme
3 tbsp gluten-free plain flour
450ml gluten-free vegetable stock
150g crème fraîche
1 x 400g tin butter beans, drained
100g spinach leaves
150g mature Cheddar cheese, grated
1 quantity chilled Rough Puff Pastry (see page 40)
1 egg, beaten

Serves 4

1 Place the butter in a large ovenproof pan over a medium heat. Once melted, add the leeks, celery and onion and fry for 2–3 minutes.

2 Add the carrots, mushrooms, peas and sweetcorn and continue to fry for another 6–8 minutes, until the veg have started to soften.

3 Sprinkle in the rosemary, thyme and flour and mix well. Pour in the vegetable stock, stir well and bring to the boil. Lower the heat and simmer for 2–3 minutes.

4 Stir in the crème fraîche, then add the butter beans, spinach and cheese. Mix well and remove from the heat.

5 Preheat the oven to 200°C/Fan 180°C/Gas Mark 6.

6 Place the chilled pastry between 2 sheets of clingfilm and roll it out to a thickness of 4mm. Don't reroll or scrunch it up at all or you'll lose the lovely layers. Place a plate slightly smaller than the diameter of the pan on the pastry and cut around it. Brush the rim of the pan with water, then carefully cover with the pastry. Cut a steam hole in the centre, then brush the top with the beaten egg. If you like, stamp small decorative shapes from the offcuts, without rerolling the pastry, and stick them to the top of the pie, before brushing again with beaten egg. Alternatively, see the tip for using pastry offcuts on page 98.

7 Bake the pie for 30 minutes, until golden brown all over. Serve hot with mashed potato and green veg.

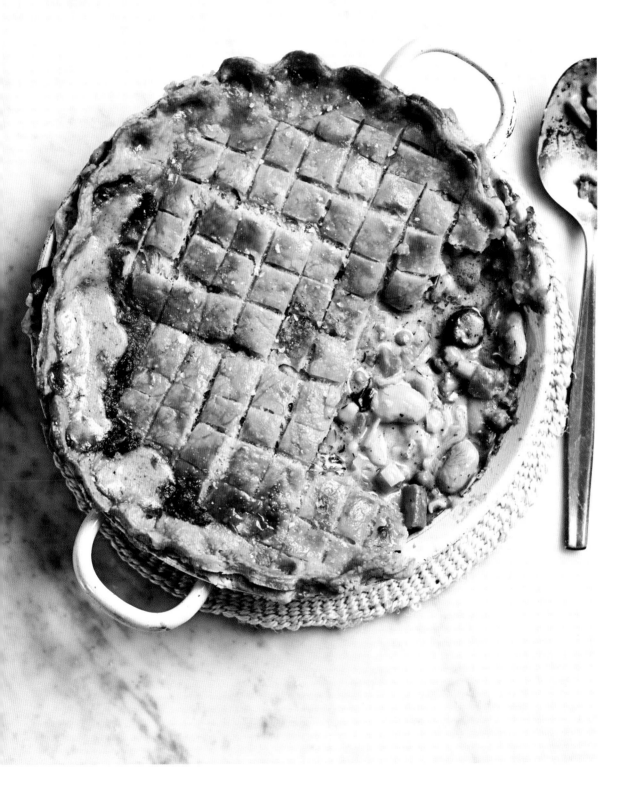

Gnocchi alla Norma

Prep: **5 minutes**
Cook: **30 minutes**

If you're wondering who Norma is and why she makes such good food, I've got a fun little factoid for you. The Italian term 'alla norma' allegedly comes from diners' enthusiastic cries of norma (masterpiece) when eating this dish. And once you've made it yourself, you'll understand why the Italians expressed their joy with such enthusiasm. It's going to become one of your weekly staples, guaranteed.

2 tbsp olive oil
2 aubergines, cut into 2cm chunks
1 tsp chilli flakes
1 tsp dried oregano
3 tsp chopped garlic
1 onion, finely chopped
2 x 400g tins chopped tomatoes
1 tbsp balsamic vinegar
50g pecorino cheese or dairy free alternative, grated
Handful of fresh basil leaves, roughly chopped
1 quantity gluten-free gnocchi (see page 34)
100ml boiling water
Salt and pepper

Serves 4

1 Place the oil in a large frying pan over a medium heat. When hot, add the aubergine, ideally in a single layer. Sprinkle with the chilli flakes, oregano and a generous seasoning of salt and pepper, mix well and fry until the aubergine has softened and started to brown a little, around 8–10 minutes. If necessary, you can fry in 2 batches, returning it all to the pan before the next step.

2 Add the garlic and onion to the pan, then stir and fry for a further 2 minutes.

3 Add the tomatoes and vinegar, mix well and bring to the boil. Lower the heat to a simmer and cook gently for 10 minutes.

4 Stir in half the cheese and three-quarters of the basil, followed by the gnocchi and boiling water. Mix gently so that the gnocchi are submerged in the sauce; you can add a little extra water if the sauce has reduced too much.

5 Cover the pan and leave simmering for 3 minutes. Stir and sprinkle with the remaining cheese and basil before serving.

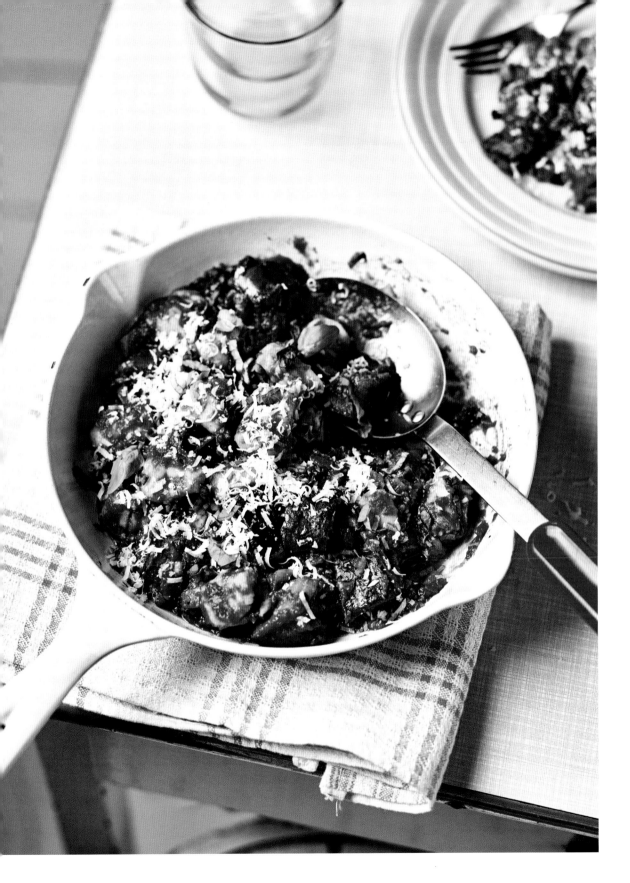

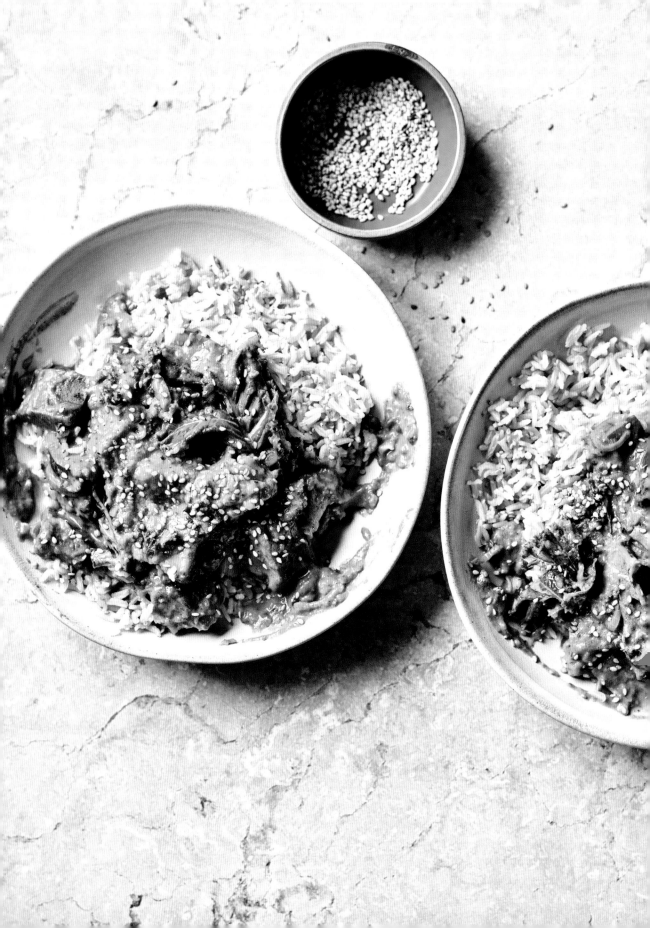

Sweet Potato & Peanut Curry

Prep: **5 minutes**
Cook: **40 minutes**

This easy vegan curry is such a nourishing meal, with soft chunks of sweet potato, flecks of vibrant kale and a spicy, satay-like sauce. You can enjoy it as a one-bowl meal on its own, serve it up with brown rice, or even portion and freeze it for an easy, microwaveable lunch. It's the multitasking meal of dreams!

1 tbsp vegetable oil
2 onions, sliced
4 tsp chopped garlic
2 tsp ginger purée
1 red chilli, deseeded and finely chopped
1 tbsp curry powder
1 tsp ground turmeric
1 tsp garam masala
1kg sweet potato, cut into 2–3cm chunks
2 tbsp tamari sauce

1 x 400ml tin coconut milk
100g peanut butter
300ml boiling water
150g chopped kale, stalks removed

To serve

Handful of freshly chopped coriander
2–3 tbsp sesame seeds or chopped peanuts

Serves 4

1   Place the oil in a large pan over a medium heat. Once hot, add the onions and fry for 6–8 minutes on a low heat, until they become translucent and lightly brown.

2   Add the garlic, ginger and chilli, mix well and fry for 1 minute. Then add the curry powder, turmeric and garam masala, stir again and fry for another 30 seconds.

3   Add the sweet potato along with the tamari and coconut milk. Mix the peanut butter and boiling water in a bowl to loosen, then add to the saucepan. Stir well, bring to the boil, then lower the heat and simmer, uncovered, for 30 minutes, stirring occasionally to prevent sticking.

4   After this time, the curry should have thickened and the sweet potatoes should be cooked through. Stir in the kale, cook for a further minute, then serve straight away, sprinkled with the fresh coriander and sesame seeds or chopped nuts. If you want to freeze this dish, leave to cool completely before portioning into tubs and freezing.

Spicy Chickpeas & Eggs

1 tbsp olive oil
150g chorizo, diced
1 red onion, finely chopped
3 tsp chopped garlic
2 tbsp harissa paste

150g red peppers from a jar,
 roughly chopped
2 x 400g tins chickpeas, drained
2 x 400g tins chopped tomatoes
4 large eggs
Chopped fresh parsley, to serve

Prep: **5 minutes**
Cook: **20 minutes**

DF

This protein-packed variation of shakshuka gives just enough of a kick to warm the cockles, and it's delicious served with chunks of freshly baked gluten-free soda bread or focaccia for dipping. I like to make a big batch of the sauce in advance, then reheat portions at various times in the week, poaching the eggs in it whenever I need a quick and easy meal. Add more harissa if you like it fiery.

Serves 4

1   Place the oil in a large frying pan over a medium heat. Once hot, add the chorizo, onion and garlic and fry for 4–5 minutes, until the chorizo starts to become crispy.

2   Add the harissa and chopped peppers to the pan, mix well and fry for another 30 seconds.

3   Pour in the chickpeas and tomatoes, stir well and bring to the boil. Lower the heat to a simmer and leave to cook for 5 minutes.

4   Using the back of a large spoon, make a well in the mixture and crack in an egg. Repeat this step for each egg. Once all 4 eggs are in the pan, cover and cook on a low heat for 3–5 minutes for a soft yolk, or 5–8 minutes for a firmer yolk.

5   Sprinkle with fresh parsley and serve with crusty gluten-free bread or toast.

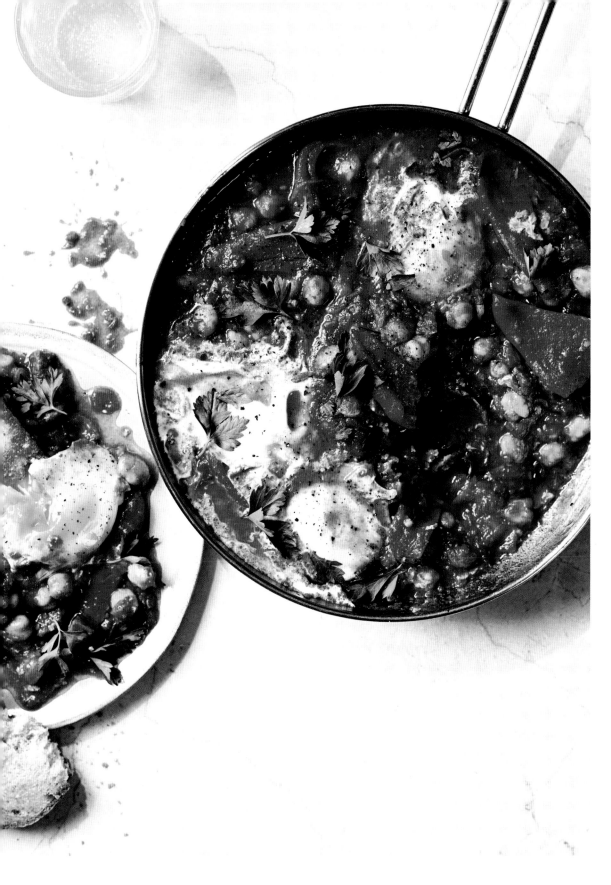

Toad-in-the-Hole

2 tbsp vegetable oil
8 gluten-free pork sausages
1 large red onion, peeled and
   cut into 8 wedges
75g gluten-free plain flour
75g cornflour
120ml milk
3 large eggs
Pinch of salt

Prep: **10 minutes**
Cook: **50 minutes**

An absolute classic, toad-in-the-hole requires minimal ingredients for the ultimate comfort dish. I like to serve mine with a good helping of mashed potato, a side of peas and lashings of gravy. You just can't beat it!

Serves 4

1   Preheat the oven to 220ºC/Fan 200ºC/Gas Mark 7.

2   Pour the oil into a 20 x 30cm non-stick roasting tray. Add the sausages, evenly spaced out, then arrange the onion wedges between them. Place in the oven for 15 minutes, shaking the tray halfway through so the sausages brown all over.

3   Meanwhile, make a batter by whisking the remaining ingredients together in a jug until smooth.

4   Once the sausages have had 15 minutes, remove the tray from the oven and pour the batter evenly over the contents. Return to the oven as quickly as possible and bake for 35 minutes, until the batter is puffy and golden. Serve hot with mash, veg and lots of gluten-free gravy.

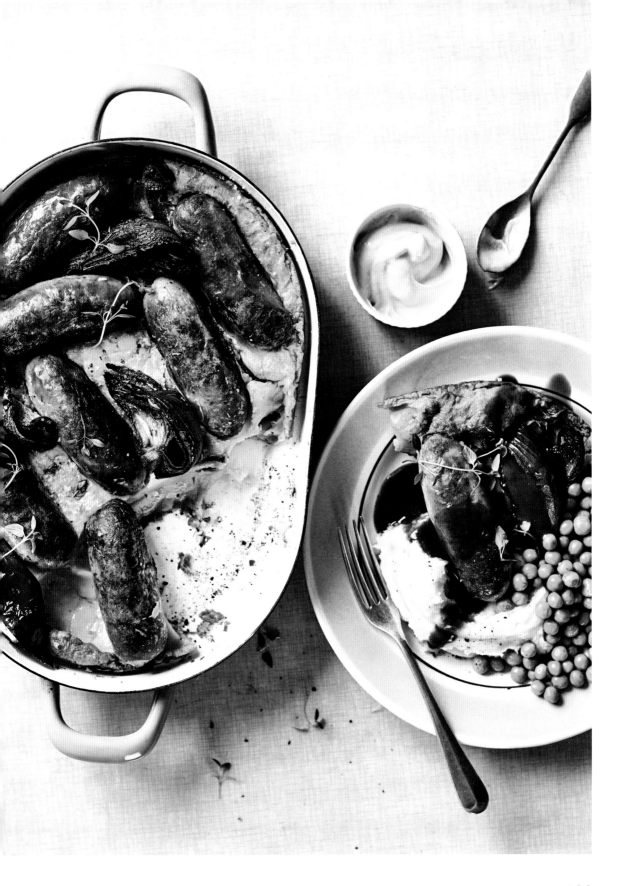

Smoky Baked Beans

1 tbsp olive oil
1 red onion, finely chopped
2 tsp chopped garlic
1 x 400g tin black beans, drained
1 x 400g tin cannellini beans, drained
500ml tomato passata
3 tsp smoked paprika
1 tbsp gluten-free Worcestershire sauce
2 tbsp maple syrup
2 tbsp tamari sauce
Gluten-free sourdough toast, to serve

Prep: **5 minutes**
Cook: **20 minutes**

EF **DF** **V**

Forget everything you thought about beans on toast, because these easy, smoky, one-pan beans are the ultimate lunch or brunch treat. They're the perfect balance of sweet and smoky, just great on a thick slab of toasted gluten-free sourdough. If you're feeling extra fancy, try adding a poached egg or even a sprinkling of cheese on top.

Serves 4

1 Place the olive oil in a pan over a medium–low heat. When hot, add the onion and garlic and fry for 2–3 minutes.

2 Add all the beans, then the passata, smoked paprika, Worcestershire sauce, maple syrup and tamari. Stir well and bring to the boil.

3 Lower the heat to a simmer, cover the pan and cook for 15 minutes, stirring once or twice, until thickened.

4 Serve hot on toasted slices of gluten-free sourdough for the ultimate beans on toast.

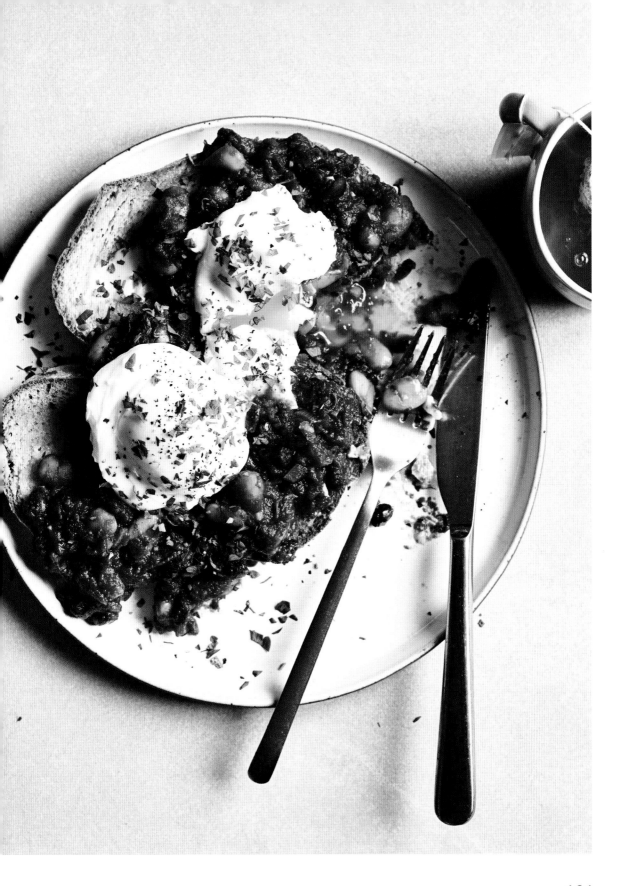

One-Pan Roast Chicken

Prep: **5 minutes**

Cook: **1 hour 40 minutes (+ 20 minutes resting)**

EF **DF**

Sometimes you really fancy a roast dinner, but the multiple pans, timings and amount of washing up can be off-putting. That's why I love this roast chicken recipe, where everything cooks together. Not only is it filled with gorgeous flavours, the juices also double as a gravy, which can be drizzled over everything when serving.

1.5kg whole chicken
800g Maris Piper potatoes
400g Chantenay carrots
200g Tenderstem broccoli
250g asparagus spears, woody ends removed

For the marinade
Juice of 2 lemons (reserve the juiced fruit)

75ml olive oil
3 tsp chopped garlic
1 tsp paprika
2 tsp dried thyme
1 tsp dried rosemary
1 tsp dried sage
1 tsp salt
½ tsp black pepper

Serves 4 ——————————

1 Preheat the oven to 200ºC/Fan 180ºC/Gas Mark 6.

2 Place the chicken in the centre of a large roasting tray.

3 Peel the potatoes and halve or quarter them so they are all about 5–7.5cm.

4 Arrange the potatoes and carrots around the chicken, keeping them spaced out and in one even layer.

5 Mix the marinade ingredients together in a bowl or jug. Stuff the squeezed lemons inside the chicken, then pour the marinade over everything in the tray, using your hands to rub it into the chicken.

6 Place the tray in the oven and roast for 30 minutes. Remove the tray, turn the potatoes and carrots over and baste the chicken with the marinade. Return to the oven for another 30 minutes.

7 Remove the tray and arrange the broccoli and asparagus around the chicken. Mix to coat them in the marinade, then baste the chicken again. Roast for another 30–40 minutes, until the juices run clear when a skewer is inserted into the thickest part of the chicken or it has an internal temperature above 75ºC.

8 Remove from the oven, cover in foil and leave to rest for 15–20 minutes before carving the chicken and plating up with the vegetables and potatoes. Drizzle any extra juices and marinade over before serving.

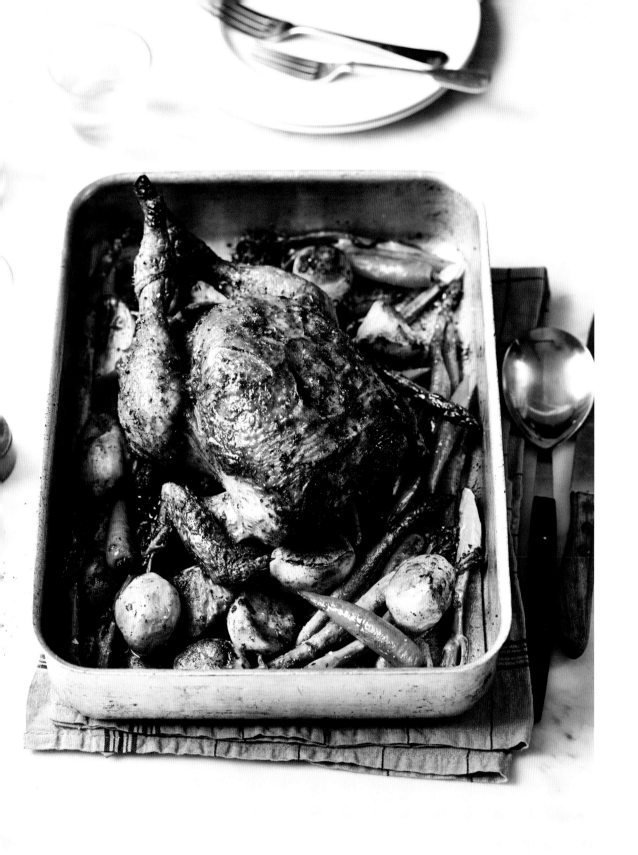

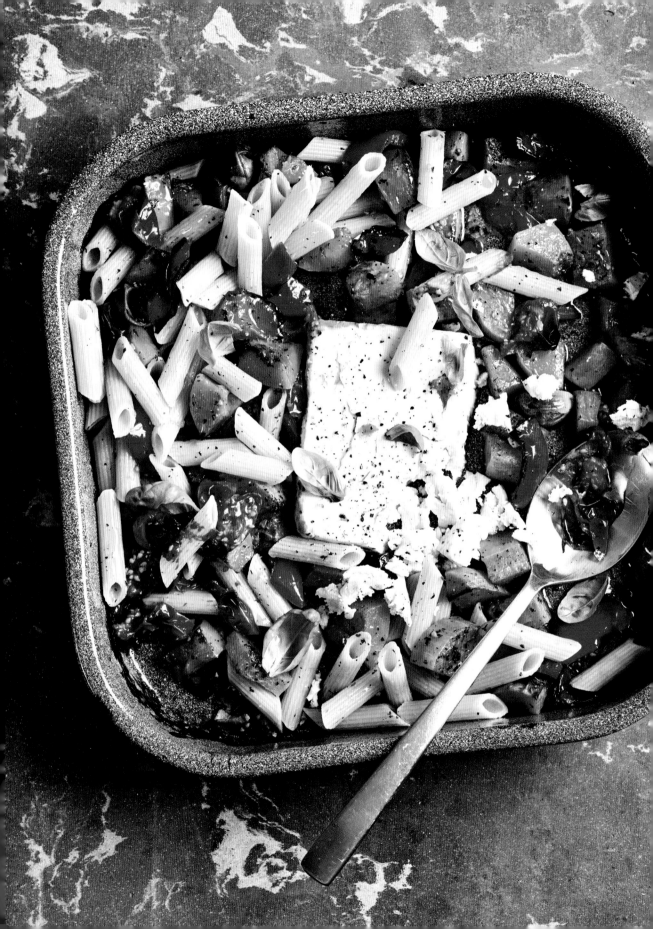

Roasted Veg & Feta Pasta

400g butternut squash, cut into
  2cm chunks
1 red pepper, deseeded and cut
  into chunks
325g baby plum tomatoes
5 garlic cloves, peeled
2 tbsp olive oil

200g feta cheese
1 tsp dried basil
1 tsp dried oregano
400g gluten-free pasta of choice
800ml gluten-free vegetable
  stock
150g Cheddar cheese, grated

Prep: **10 minutes**
Cook: **1 hour 5 minutes**

Did you know that baking feta
turns it into the creamiest pasta
sauce? When you mix this sauce
with a medley of beautifully roasted
vegetables, it becomes a super
dinner that is both decadent and
nutrient-packed. I love how easy this
dish is to make – no need for extra
washing up, as the pasta cooks in
the sauce, all in one pan.

Serves 4

1 Preheat the oven to 200ºC/Fan 180ºC/Gas Mark 6.

2 Place the squash, red pepper, tomatoes and garlic cloves in a
large roasting tray and drizzle over the olive oil. Sprinkle over
the basil and oregano and toss together.

3 Create a space in the middle of the tray and nestle the block
of feta there. Place in the oven for 35 minutes, turning the veg
halfway through, but being careful not to break up the feta.

4 When the baking time is up, stir the softened feta into the
vegetables, then roughly 'mush' up the veg using a potato
masher or fork. You want a semi-smooth texture – some
lumps of veg are fine.

5 Stir in the uncooked pasta, then pour in the stock, ensuring
the pasta is all submerged. Return to the oven for 10 minutes,
then stir well and sprinkle over the grated cheese. Return
to the oven for another 10–15 minutes, until the cheese is
melted and golden and the pasta has cooked through.
Serve hot.

Sausage & Sweet Potato Traybake

Prep: **5 minutes**
Cook: **40 minutes**

EF   **DF**

The combination of honey and mustard is a classic that just works so well with sausages. And when it comes to a flavour-packed dinner, it doesn't get much easier than this. It includes lots of veg, but feel free to add any others you love – chunks of courgette, aubergine or even cherry tomatoes would also work well.

750g sweet potato, peeled and cut into 5cm chunks
1 red pepper, deseeded and cut into 5cm chunks
1 large red onion, cut into wedges
1 tbsp olive oil
8 gluten-free pork sausages
200g Tenderstem broccoli
3 tbsp runny honey
2 tbsp wholegrain mustard
Salt and pepper

Serves 4 _____

1   Preheat the oven to 220°C/Fan 200°C/Gas Mark 7.

2   Place the sweet potato, red pepper and onion in a large, non-stick roasting tray. Drizzle with the olive oil, generously season with salt and pepper, then toss to coat.

3   Nestle the sausages among the vegetables, trying to space things evenly, then roast for 20 minutes.

4   Remove the tray from the oven and use a large spoon to turn the sausages and veg over. Scatter the broccoli evenly across the tray, then return it to the oven for another 15 minutes.

5   Mix the honey and mustard together in a bowl. Remove the tray from the oven and drizzle the dressing over the contents, making sure everything is coated. Return to the oven for another 5 minutes, then serve.

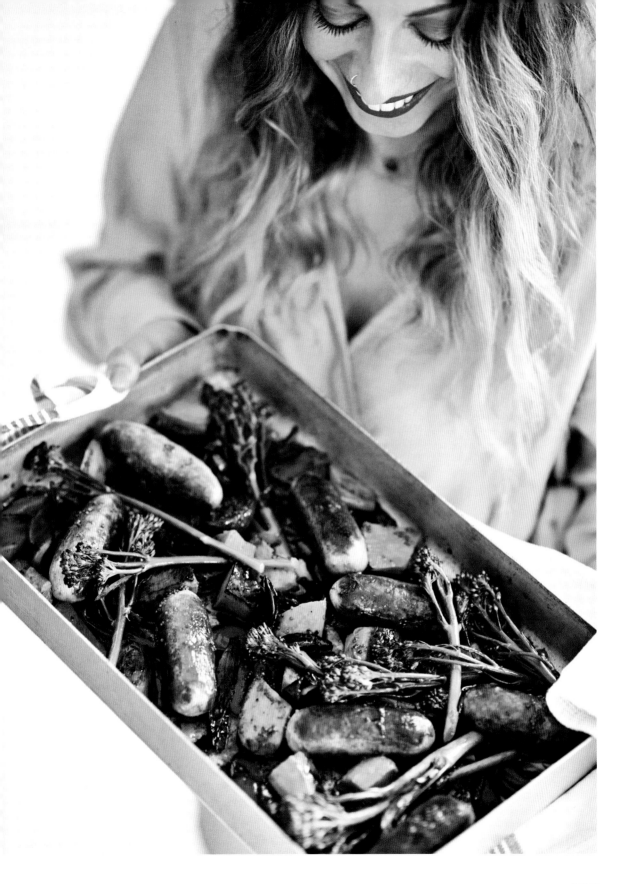

Garlicky Lemon Salmon & Potatoes

1kg baby potatoes
2 tbsp olive oil
4 tbsp gluten-free vegetable
  stock
4 tsp chopped garlic
Juice of 1 lemon

1 tbsp sriracha sauce
4 salmon fillets
200g Tenderstem broccoli
200g green beans, trimmed
Lemon slices (optional)
Sea salt flakes

Prep: **5 minutes**
Cook: **35 minutes**

EF **DF**

Sometimes you just need a good, nourishing meal that can be chucked in the oven without much thought, so this is my go-to post-workout meal. It's ideal partly because the garlicky sauce with a hint of spice and tang provides the best flavours for the salmon and vegetables, and partly because it cooks in the exact time it takes me to shower and dry my hair.

Serves 4

1 Preheat the oven to 220ºC/Fan 200ºC/Gas Mark 7.

2 Cut the potatoes into halves or quarters, depending on size. They should all be roughly the same. Place in a roasting tray and drizzle with half the olive oil. Add a pinch of sea salt and toss to coat the potatoes. Roast for 20 minutes, turning them halfway through.

3 Meanwhile, put the stock in a small bowl with the garlic, lemon juice, sriracha and remaining olive oil, and mix together.

4 When the potatoes are done, push them to the sides of the tray and place the salmon fillets, skin-side down, in the middle, spacing them slightly apart. Arrange the broccoli and green beans around the salmon and potatoes, then drizzle the stock mixture over everything. Top the salmon with some lemon slices, if you like, then return the tray to the oven for another 15 minutes.

5 Once the salmon is cooked through and beautifully flaky, serve straight away.

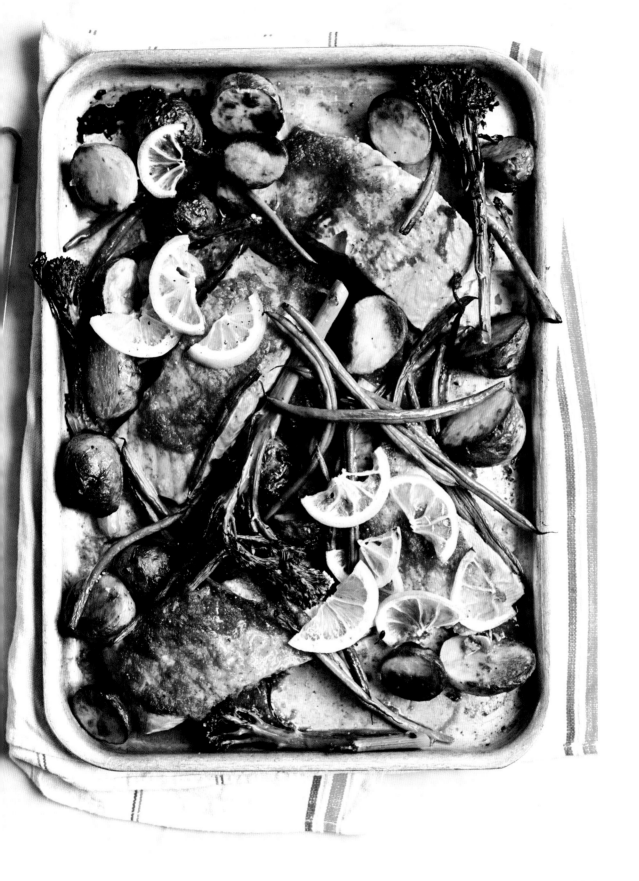

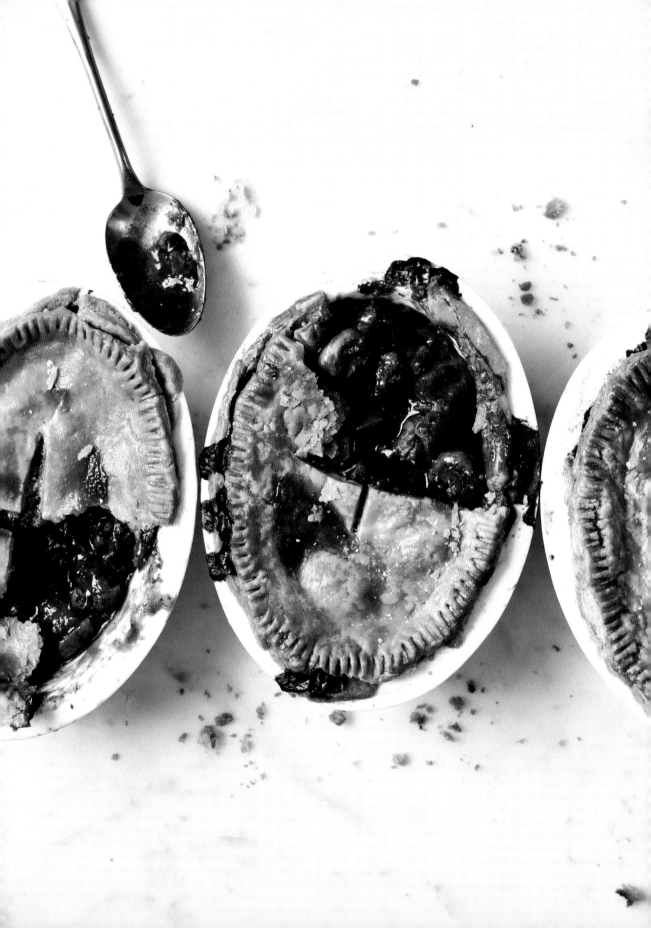

WEEKEND WARMERS

Just because something takes a long time to cook, it doesn't mean it has to involve a lot of effort. Plus, as a famous gluten-containing drinks brand once said, 'Good things come to those who wait'. These recipes tend to use cheaper cuts of meat or ingredients that benefit from slow cooking, often making them a more affordable option. You'll need an ovenproof casserole dish that can also be used on the hob, or a slow cooker – both will give great results.

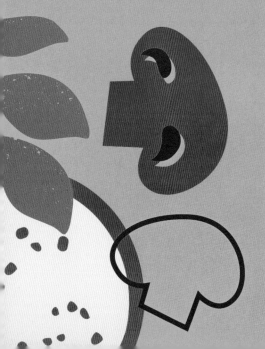

'Devon Maid' Pork & Cider Casserole

1 tbsp olive oil
600g pork shoulder, cut into 5–7½cm chunks
30g unsalted butter or dairy-free alternative
125g smoked bacon lardons
1 leek, sliced
1 onion, chopped
300g Chantenay carrots
2 tsp dried sage
3 tbsp gluten-free plain flour
1 gluten-free chicken stock cube dissolved in 200ml boiling water
500ml dry cider
Salt and pepper

Prep: **30 minutes**
Cook: **2½ hours**

EF   DFO

I'm proud of being a Devon girl, and, if there's one ingredient that basically runs in my blood, it's cider. So naturally, one of the recipes in this book had to be my hearty pork and cider casserole. The pork shoulder falls apart beautifully when slow-cooked and the cider adds a hint of sweetness to this classic winter warmer. I absolutely love a Chantenay carrot, but you can just chop ordinary carrots into chunks if you don't want to be as fancy-pants as me.

Serves 4

1   Preheat the oven to 160°C/Fan 140°C/Gas Mark 3.

2   Place the olive oil in a large frying pan over a high heat. Once hot, fry the pork – you might need to do this in batches – turning until it's browned on all sides. Set to one side.

3   Place the butter in a large flameproof casserole dish over a medium heat. Once melted, add the lardons, leek, onion and carrots. Fry for 6–8 minutes, until softened.

4   Add the seared pork to the pan, sprinkle the sage and flour over everything and mix well.

5   Pour the stock into the casserole dish, along with the cider. Generously season with salt and pepper and stir well, scraping up any bits stuck to the bottom of the pan. Bring to the boil, cover with a lid and place in the oven for 2½ hours. Once done, stir well and serve with mashed potatoes.

▶▶ SLOW COOKER SWAP

Follow the recipe to the end of step 4, then add everything to the slow cooker. Cook on high for 3–4 hours, or low for 6–8 hours.

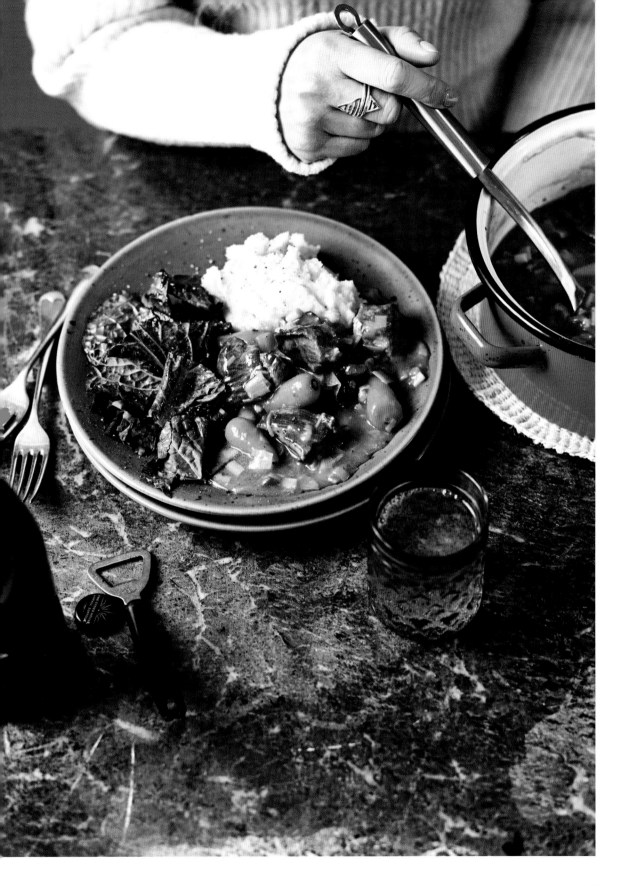

Hearty Beef Stew

Prep: **20 minutes**
Cook: **3 hours**

25g butter or dairy-free
  alternative
2 tbsp gluten-free plain flour
500g diced beef shin
100g bacon lardons
1 onion, chopped
3 large carrots (about 500g),
  cut into chunks
200g mushrooms, halved

150ml red wine
500ml hot water
2 bay leaves
2 tsp dried thyme
1 tsp dried rosemary
1 gluten-free beef stock pot
1 tbsp tomato purée
1 tbsp gluten-free
  Worcestershire sauce

Nothing beats a rich stew filled with big flavours – not to mention the incredible smells that will fill your house as it cooks. This recipe uses red wine and rich beef stock to create a dreamy stew that is full of flavour. Using beef shin keeps the cost down, and it becomes beautifully tender when cooked slowly. This is what lazy Sunday afternoons were made for.

Serves 4

1   Preheat the oven to 180°C/Fan 160°C/Gas Mark 4.

2   Heat the butter in a large, flameproof casserole dish over a medium heat. Put the flour on a large plate or in a large freezer bag, add the beef and turn or shake to coat well. Add to the pan along with the bacon lardons and fry for 4–5 minutes, until the beef has browned on all sides. Transfer to a clean plate.

3   Add the onion, carrot and mushrooms to the pan and fry for 4–5 minutes over a medium heat, until the veg start to soften and brown.

4   Return the beef, bacon and any juices to the pan, then add all the remaining ingredients. Stir well, bring to the boil, then turn off the heat. Cover with a lid and cook in the oven for 3 hours, until the meat falls apart easily.

▶▶ SLOW COOKER **SWAP**

After frying off the beef and bacon, place them in the slow cooker. Add the fried vegetables, followed by the remaining ingredients. Mix well and cook on high for 4–5 hours, or low for 7–8 hours.

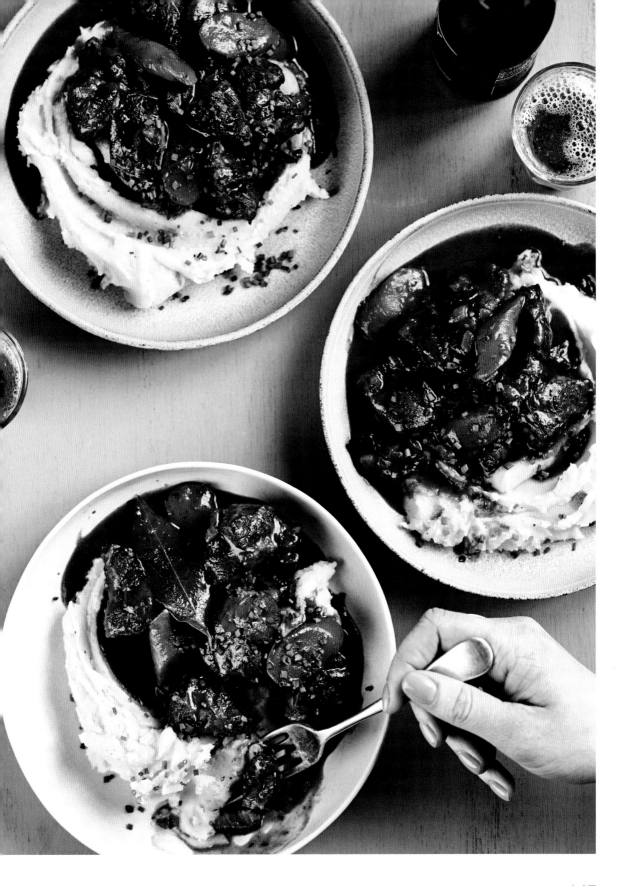

Chicken Casserole with Suet Dumplings

Prep: **30 minutes**
Cook: **1 hour**

To me, a chicken casserole is the ultimate winter comfort food, but having to be gluten free means I miss out on the dumplings. Not any more! Some supermarket suet is gluten free, and it's worth hunting it down to make these squidgy and delicious dumplings, which cook to perfection in a sauce packed with flavour. I always keep some of this casserole in the freezer for emergencies.

TOP TIP

Can't get hold of any gluten-free suet? Grab some cold, unsalted butter – the same quantity as specified above – then grate and use it in the same way as the suet. It will work just as well.

SLOW COOKER SWAP

Add the browned chicken and veg to the slow cooker after step 5 (the browning is crucial for flavour). Cook on high for 3–4 hours, or low for 6 hours, adding the dumplings for the final hour of cooking.

2 tbsp plain gluten-free flour
4 large skinless chicken thigh fillets
2 tbsp olive oil
4 rashers streaky bacon, chopped
2 large carrots, chopped into 2cm chunks
1 large onion, finely chopped
1 tbsp Dijon mustard
2 tsp dried thyme
1 tsp dried sage
500ml gluten-free chicken stock
185ml white wine
Salt and pepper

For the dumplings
150g gluten-free plain flour
2 tsp baking powder
75g gluten-free vegetable suet
120ml cold water

Serves 4

1. Preheat the oven to 180°C/Fan 160°C/Gas Mark 4.

2. Place the 2 tablespoons of flour on a large plate or in tub and season with salt and pepper. Add the chicken fillets and turn or shake to coat well.

3. Add half the olive oil to a large flameproof casserole dish over a high heat. Once hot, fry the fillets for 7–8 minutes, turning halfway through, until they have nicely browned. Transfer them to a clean plate.

4. Lower the heat under the casserole dish to medium and add the remaining olive oil, the bacon, carrots and onion and sauté, with the lid on, for 7–8 minutes, stirring occasionally.

5. Return the fried chicken to the dish, then add the mustard, dried herbs, stock and wine. Stir well, bring to a simmer, then cover and place in the oven for 35 minutes.

6. Meanwhile, mix the dumpling ingredients together in a bowl until they form a sticky dough. Cover with a tea towel and leave for 10–15 minutes.

7. When the casserole has had 35 minutes, remove the pan from the oven and use your hands to divide the dumpling mixture into 8–10 equal pieces. Roll them into balls and place in the casserole so they are half-submerged in the sauce.

8. Replace the lid and return the dish to the oven for another 20 minutes. Remove the lid and cook for a further 5 minutes. Serve hot with lots of green veg.

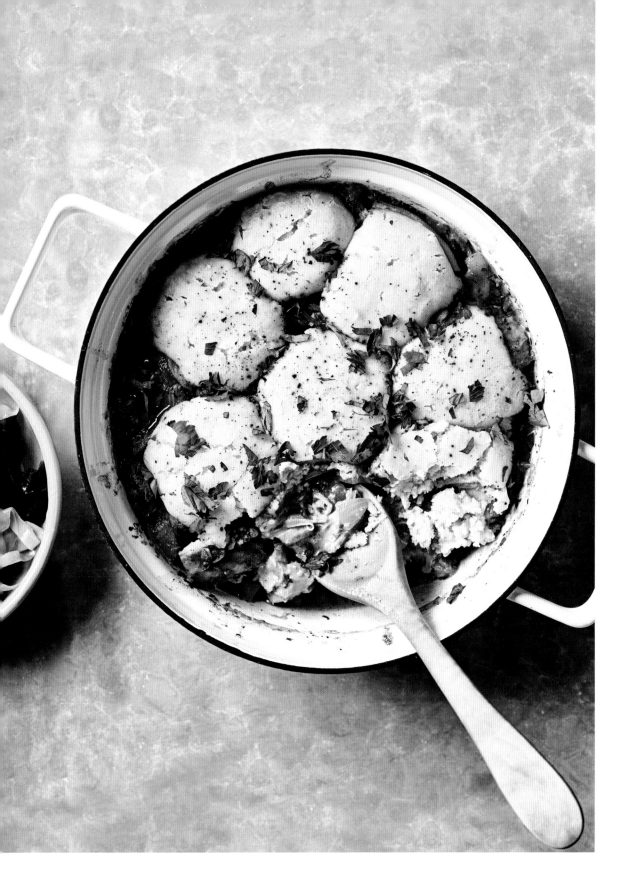

Gammon with Ginger Beer Glaze

Prep: **20 minutes**
Cook: **2 hours**

EF **DF**

Slow cooking gammon in ginger beer is, in my opinion, the best and only way to cook it. The joint makes a regular appearance at our Christmas dinner, with the glaze adding the perfect finishing touch. The recipe here includes roasted root vegetables and a fresh parsley sauce, which turn it into a delicious alternative to a traditional Sunday lunch. If you like, you can boil the ham a day in advance, then glaze it and finish in the oven for 30–35 minutes before serving.

TOP TIP

Freeze any uneaten ham in slices, or chopped into small cubes for using in my Chicken, Ham & Leek Puff Pie (see page 98).

1.3kg gammon joint
1 onion, peeled and quartered
1 carrot, roughly chopped into chunks
2 whole garlic cloves, peeled
1.5 litres non-diet ginger beer
1 tbsp wholegrain mustard
1 tbsp honey
1 tbsp light brown sugar

For the roasted veg
250g sweet potatoes
250g white potatoes
250g carrots
200g parsnips
200g beetroot
2 tbsp olive oil
Sea salt flakes
1 tsp dried thyme

For the parsley sauce
1 quantity White Sauce (see page 32)
Large handful of fresh parsley, chopped

Serves 4

1 Place the gammon in a snug-fitting flameproof casserole dish and arrange the onion, carrot and garlic cloves around it. Reserve 100ml of the ginger beer, then pour the rest over the joint. It should be completely covered, so top up with water if necessary. Bring to the boil, cover with a lid and adjust the heat to a low, rolling boil. Leave for 1½ hours, checking it occasionally. If the liquid reduces too much, top up with a little extra water, or ginger beer if you have any to spare.

2 When the joint has cooked for just over an hour, chop the unpeeled vegetables into 5cm chunks (the skin adds extra goodness).

3 Preheat the oven to 200°C/Fan 180°C/Gas Mark 6.

4 Place the prepared veg in a large roasting tray and sprinkle with the oil, thyme and a good pinch of sea salt flakes. Toss well, then roast for 20 minutes.

5 Once the gammon is cooked, use tongs to transfer it to a plate, then discard the cooking liquid and vegetables.

6 To make the glaze, place the reserved ginger beer in a small saucepan, add the mustard, honey and sugar, and bring to the boil. Continue boiling for 5 minutes, until it has reduced to a syrupy consistency.

7 Increase the oven temperature to 220°C/Fan 200°C/Gas Mark 7.

8 Using a sharp knife, remove any skin from the gammon, leaving a layer of fat, then score the fat in a diamond pattern.

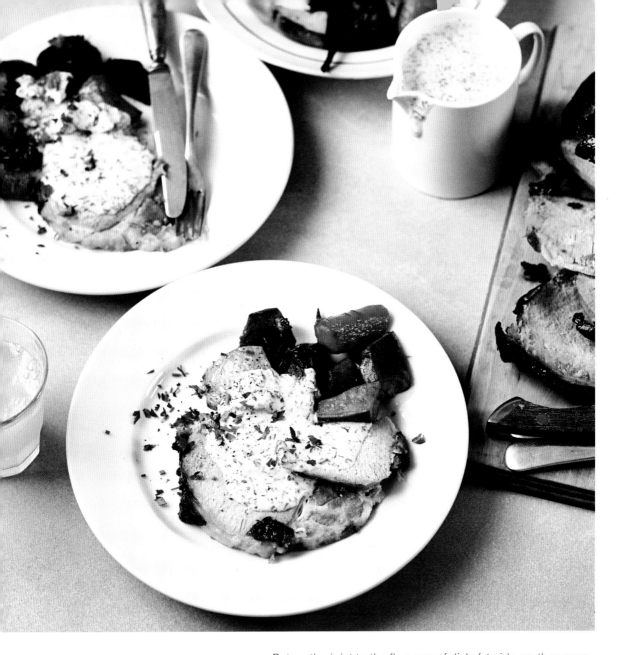

Return the joint to the flameproof dish, fat-side up, then pour the glaze over it. Place in the oven for 20–25 minutes, until the glaze has caramelised.

SLOW COOKER SWAP

Place the gammon and vegetables in the slow cooker, cover with the ginger beer and cook on high for 3–4 hours, or low for 6–8 hours. Score the joint and finish in the oven as described in step 8.

9 Stir and turn the roasting vegetables and cook for a further 25–30 minutes, until they have started to brown around the edges and you can easily push a dinner knife through the centre of the biggest chunk.

10 When the gammon and vegetables are ready, warm the white sauce and stir in the chopped parsley. Slice the ham and serve with a good helping of the roasted veg and a smothering of parsley sauce.

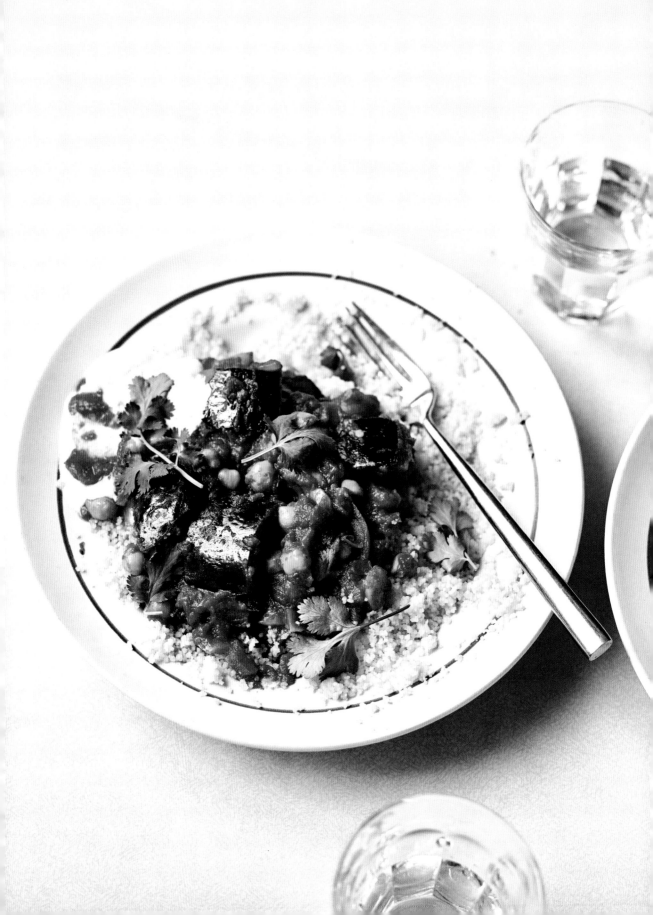

Aubergine Tagine

Prep: **15 minutes**
Cook: **1 hour**

3 tbsp olive oil
2 aubergines, cut into 2.5cm chunks
1 red onion, finely diced
3 tsp chopped garlic
1 red pepper, deseeded and chopped
1 yellow pepper, deseeded and chopped
1 x 400g tin chickpeas, drained
2 tbsp ras el hanout
2 x 400g tins chopped tomatoes
200ml gluten-free vegetable stock
100g dried apricots, halved
Handful of fresh coriander leaves, for sprinkling (optional)

I love the rich, fiery flavours of a Moroccan-style tagine, and this vegan version is a hearty dish that even meat-eaters will love. You can find ras el hanout spice mixture in most supermarkets, and any you don't use in this recipe can be used as a rub for various meats. If you can find gluten-free couscous, you'll get the authentic style of this dish; if not, quinoa or rice work very well too. Be warned – this tagine packs a fiery punch!

Serves 4

1 Preheat the oven to 200ºC/Fan 180ºC/Gas Mark 6.

2 Place a flameproof tagine or casserole dish over a medium-low heat and add the oil. Once hot, add the aubergine and fry for 8–10 minutes, until browned on all sides.

3 Stir in the onion and garlic and fry for 2–3 minutes, stirring well, then add the peppers and fry for another 2–3 minutes.

4 Add the chickpeas to the pan, sprinkle over the ras el hanout and stir well, frying for another 30 seconds.

5 Add the tomatoes, stock and apricots, mix well and bring to the boil. Cover with a lid and place in the oven for 30 minutes. Stir well and return to the oven, without a lid, for another 10–15 minutes. Meanwhile, make the couscous, quinoa or rice.

6 Remove the tagine from the oven, mix well and sprinkle with fresh coriander if you wish.

7 Serve with gluten-free couscous, quinoa or rice.

TOP TIP

This tagine is designed to be pretty spicy, so, if you like things milder, add just half the ras el hanout listed above. Alternatively, add some dollops of Greek or dairy-free yoghurt to the finished dish.

SLOW COOKER SWAP

Follow steps 2–4 above, then transfer the mixture to the slow cooker and add all the remaining ingredients. Cook for 2–3 hours on high, or 4–5 hours on low.

Next Level Lasagne

Prep: **20 minutes**
Cook: **1 hour 40 minutes**

EF

With layers of rich ragu and oozing cheese sauce, this is a lasagne unlike any you've had before. The star of the show is the meaty sauce made from beef mince and pork sausage-meat, which is slow-cooked and oh, so delicious. To save time on the day you want to serve it, you can make the separate sauces the day before. In fact, I always make a double batch so I have some in the freezer for next time I get a lasagne craving.

1 quantity gluten-free Fresh Pasta dough (see page 36), cut into 16 lasagne sheets

For the ragu
1 tbsp olive oil
1 onion, finely chopped
1 celery stick, finely chopped
1 carrot, finely chopped
2 tsp chopped garlic
3 gluten-free pork sausages
250g beef mince
1 tsp dried thyme
1 tsp dried oregano
1 tsp dried rosemary
250ml gluten-free beef stock

125ml red wine
1 x 400g tin chopped tomatoes
2 tbsp tomato purée

For the cheese sauce
50g unsalted butter
50g gluten-free plain flour
500ml milk
150g mature Cheddar cheese, grated
50g mozzarella cheese, grated
1 tbsp grated Parmesan cheese, plus extra for sprinkling
Salt and pepper

Serves 4

1. To make the ragu, place the olive oil in a large saucepan over a medium heat. Add the onion, celery, carrot and garlic, mix well and fry on a low heat for 6–7 minutes, until the vegetables have started to soften.

2. Remove the skins from the sausages and roughly chop the sausage-meat. Once the veg has softened, turn the heat up to medium–high and add the beef mince and sausage-meat. Use a spatula to break up the meat, while frying for 7–8 minutes, until it has browned all over.

3. Add the herbs, stock, wine, tomatoes and tomato purée and mix well. Bring to the boil, then lower the heat to a simmer, and cook uncovered for 45 minutes, stirring occasionally. The ragu should thicken up nicely. Taste and adjust the seasoning if necessary – I find the stock cube usually adds enough salt. If making the ragu in advance, cool completely at this point and store in the fridge until needed.

4. To make the cheese sauce, melt the butter in a large pan over a low heat, then whisk in the flour to form a thick paste. Continue cooking and stirring for about 30–60 seconds to ensure it doesn't stick. Pour in about 100ml of the milk and stir constantly over the heat until it forms a smooth, thick paste. Continue adding the milk 100ml at a time, stirring constantly between each addition, until you have a smooth white sauce. Add the grated cheeses and stir until melted.

5. When you're ready to construct the lasagne, preheat the oven to 200°C/Fan 180°C/Gas Mark 6. Lay out the lasagne sheets.

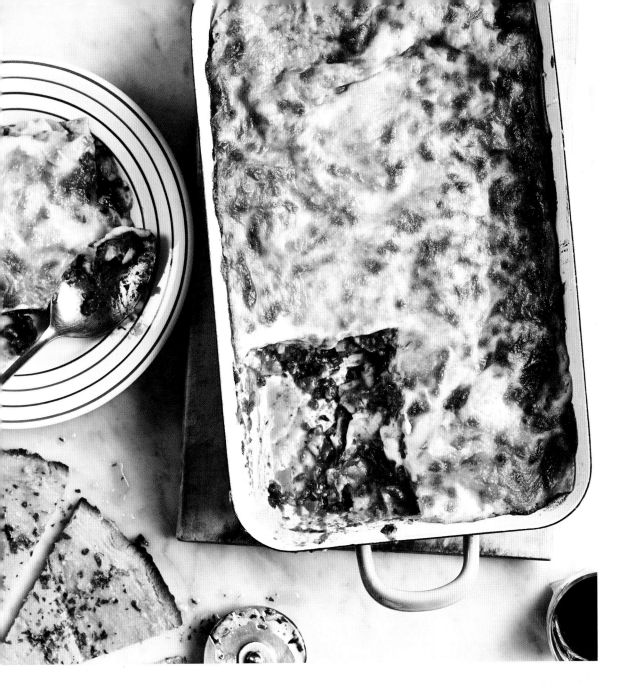

 SLOW COOKER SWAP

Brown the vegetables, sausage-meat and mince as described above, then transfer to the slow cooker and add all the remaining ragu ingredients. Cook on high for 3-4 hours, or low for 6-8 hours.

6 Spoon a third of the ragu into a 20 x 30cm baking dish and spread evenly. Cover with some of the lasagne sheets, overlapping them slightly, then spoon over a third of the cheese sauce, spreading it out to the edges. Cover with more lasagne sheets as before, then repeat the layers until you have used up everything, finishing with a layer of cheese sauce.

7 Sprinkle extra grated Parmesan on top and bake for 40-45 minutes, until golden and bubbling. Serve straight away with gluten-free garlic pizza bread (see page 215).

Steak & Mushroom Pie

Prep: **30 minutes**
Cook: **3½ hours**

A hearty pie is a thing of beauty, and the steak and mushroom filling here uses gluten-free ale, or stout, for a really rich flavour. This is the perfect Sunday dinner, served hot with lashings of gluten-free beef gravy and a big dollop of mashed potato. And if there are any leftovers, you can easily freeze them for a simple dinner another night.

TOP TIP ▷▷▷▷▷▷

Want to make individual pies instead of a large one? Simply use 4 x 12cm pie dishes and bake for 30–35 minutes.

1 quantity chilled Shortcrust
   Pastry (see page 39)
Gluten-free plain flour,
   for dusting
1 egg, beaten

For the filling
30g dried porcini mushrooms
300ml boiling water
500g diced beef shin
3 tbsp gluten-free plain flour
50g unsalted butter
330ml gluten-free ale or stout
1 onion, finely diced
2 carrots, halved lengthways,
   then cut into small chunks
250g baby chestnut mushrooms
1 tbsp chopped fresh thyme
1 tbsp chopped fresh rosemary
1 tbsp tomato purée
1 tbsp gluten-free
   Worcestershire sauce
1 gluten-free beef stock pot
Salt and pepper

Serves 4

1 Preheat the oven to 180°C/Fan 160°C/Gas Mark 4. Start by making the filling.

2 Put the dried mushrooms in a bowl, cover with the boiling water and leave to sit for 20 minutes.

3 Place the flour on a large plate or in a tub and generously season with salt and pepper. Add the beef and turn or shake until fully coated.

4 Melt half the butter in a large flameproof casserole dish over a medium–high heat. Once hot, add the beef and any excess flour, and fry for 4–5 minutes, until the meat is brown on all sides. Transfer to a plate.

5 Add a splash of the ale to the pan and use a spoon or spatula to scrape up any bits stuck to the bottom. Pour this liquid onto the same plate as the beef.

6 Return the pan to the heat and melt the remaining butter. Add the onion, carrots and chestnut mushrooms and fry for 4–5 minutes, until beginning to soften.

7 Take the pan off the heat and add the beef and juices, the porcini mushrooms and their liquid, the remaining ale, the herbs, tomato purée, Worcestershire sauce and stock pot. Mix well, cover with a lid and place in the oven for 2 hours, until the beef is tender and falls apart easily. When done, set aside until cooled to room temperature. If necessary, it can be left overnight in the fridge.

8 When you're ready to assemble the pie, preheat the oven to 200°C/Fan 180°C/Gas Mark 6.

9   Place the chilled pastry on a floured work surface and knead until it is malleable. At that point, roll it out to a thickness of 4mm, using a little more flour if necessary to stop it sticking.

10 Use your rolling pin to lift the pastry over a 23cm pie dish, then gently press it into place, remembering to cover the lip too. Trim off the excess and set aside. Prick the bottom of the pastry case with a fork. Spoon the cooled filling into the dish, spreading it evenly.

11 Gather the leftover pastry into a ball and roll it into a circle about 4mm thick and slightly larger than the diameter of the dish.

12 Brush the lip of the pastry case with beaten egg, then gently lay the pastry lid over the top. Press the edges together with your fingers, then trim with a knife. Use a fork to press all around the rim.

13 Cut a steam hole in the top of the pie, then brush the surface with the beaten egg. If you like, reroll any remnants of pastry and cut shapes from them to decorate your pie. Brush again with beaten egg.

14 Place the pie in the oven for 45–60 minutes, until golden and bubbling. Serve straight away.

 SLOW COOKER SWAP

Follow the recipe up to step 7, then place everything in the slow cooker for 3–4 hours on high, or 6–8 hours on low. If the mixture becomes too watery, you can thicken it up by stirring 1 tablespoon cornflour mixed with 2 tablespoons cold water into the mixture while it's still hot.

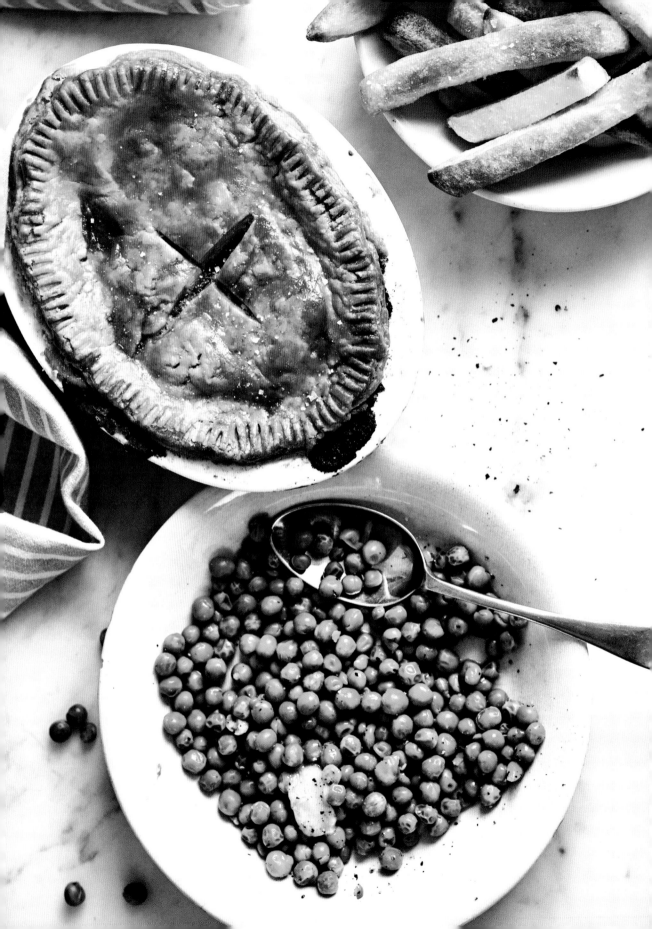

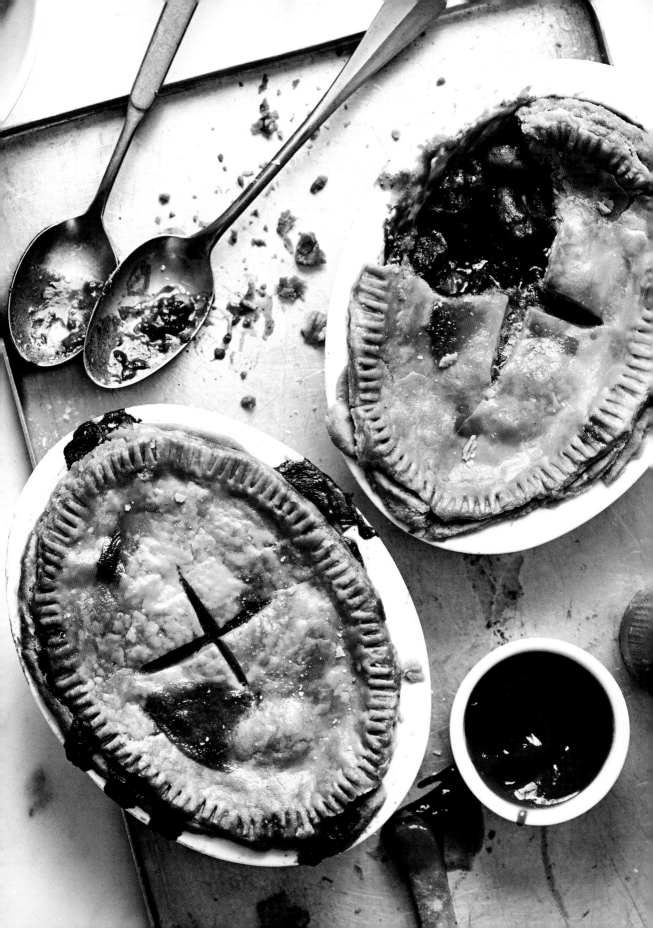

Beef Brisket with Red Wine Gravy

1kg beef brisket, at room temperature (takes at least 30 minutes)
1 tbsp olive oil
2 onions, quartered
6 garlic cloves, peeled
3 sprigs of fresh thyme
1 carrot, cut into rough chunks
150ml red wine
1 tbsp gluten-free Worcestershire sauce
1 gluten-free beef stock cube dissolved in 200ml boiling water
1½ tbsp cornflour mixed with 1–2 tbsp cold water
Salt and pepper

Prep: **15 minutes**
Cook: **4¾ hours**

EF   **DF**

Brisket is a comparatively cheap cut of meat that becomes beautifully tender when slow-cooked. Here it stews in a flavour-filled stock that can be thickened and served as gravy – in this case, completely gluten free. I like to serve the joint with green beans and either mashed or roasted potatoes for a tasty Sunday lunch.

Serves 4 _____

1   Preheat the oven to 140°C/Fan 120°C/Gas Mark 1.

2   Place the oil in a large, ovenproof casserole dish over a high heat. Once hot, season the brisket generously with salt and pepper, then sear in the pan until brown on all sides. Turn off the heat.

3   Arrange the onions, garlic, thyme and carrot around the beef, then add the wine, Worcestershire sauce and stock. The beef should be at least half-submerged. If not, top up with some extra beef stock or hot water.

4   Cover with a lid and place in the oven for 4½ hours, turning the beef over at least once during this time.

5   Transfer the cooked beef to a plate, cover with foil and leave to rest for 30 minutes.

6   To make the gravy, use a potato masher to roughly mash the vegetables in the remaining liquid. Strain through a sieve into a jug, discarding the veg. Pour the liquid back into the pan.

7   Place the pan over a medium–high heat and bring to the boil. Stir in the cornflour slurry and simmer for 1–2 minutes, until nicely thickened.

8   Once the meat has rested, slice the beef and serve with chipped potatoes, greens and the lovely red wine gravy.

 SLOW COOKER SWAP

Sear the beef as described, then arrange in the slow cooker as per step 3. Cook on high for 4–5 hours, or low for 8 hours. Once cooked, follow steps 5–8 to complete the dish.

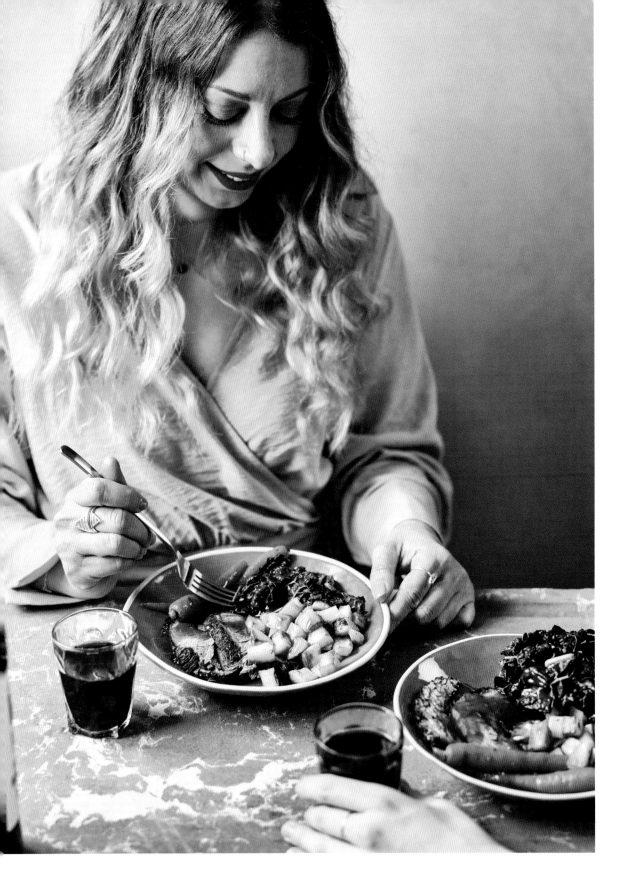

Mexican Pulled Chicken

1 tsp olive oil
1 onion, finely chopped
1 x 400g tin chopped tomatoes
600g skinless and boneless
   chicken thigh fillets

For the marinade
2 tbsp olive oil
1 red chilli, deseeded and finely
   chopped
1 tbsp smoked paprika
1 tsp ground cumin
½ tsp cayenne pepper
1 tsp garlic granules
Juice of 1 lime
Salt and pepper

Prep: **10 minutes**
(+ 24 hours to marinate)

Cook: **1 hour 20 minutes**

EF **DF**

If you love Mexican food and want a real 'hands off' approach, this pulled chicken is perfect. The meat is cooked in a zingy and spicy marinade with minimal effort. I love batch-cooking this pulled chicken as part of my meal prep, using it in tacos, burritos, wraps and salads, or served with a pouch of microwave rice for those lazy nights. While you can get away with marinating the chicken for an hour or two, it's far better if you leave it in the fridge overnight so that it really absorbs all the lovely flavours in the marinade.

 SLOW COOKER SWAP

Marinade the meat as in step 1, then add to the slow cooker along with all the other ingredients. You can fry the onions first if you like, but it's not essential. Cook on high for 3–4 hours, or low for 6–8 hours.

Serves 4

1 Combine all the marinade ingredients in a large bowl, then add the chicken and toss to coat. Cover and leave in the fridge for at least 1–2 hours, but ideally overnight.

2 When you're ready to cook, preheat the oven to 180°C/160°C Fan/Gas Mark 4.

3 Place the olive oil in a large, flameproof casserole dish over a medium–low heat. Once hot, add the onions and fry gently for 6–8 minutes, until softened. Add the tomatoes and mix well, then take off the heat.

4 Add the chicken to the dish, along with as much marinade as possible. Mix well so the chicken is submerged in the tomatoes.

5 Place a sheet of foil over the pan, cover with a lid to make a tight seal. Place in the oven for 1 hour, then remove and increase the temperature to 200°C/Fan 180°C/Gas Mark 6. Use tongs to transfer the chicken to a chopping board, then use 2 forks to pull it apart.

6 Once the meat is shredded, return it to the casserole dish, stir well, then replace in the oven, uncovered, for another 15 minutes.

7 Serve in gluten-free tacos or burritos or with rice and salad.

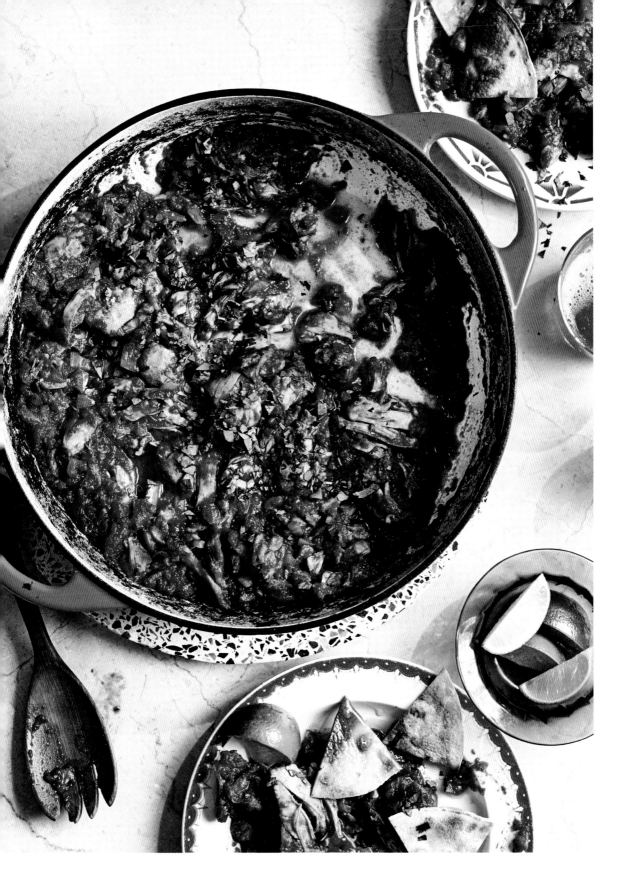

Butternut Squash & Stilton Wellington

Prep: **30 minutes**
Cook: **1 hour**

Sometimes an occasion calls for a grand centrepiece, and this easy Wellington recipe fits the bill. It not only looks stunning, but is gluten free and vegetarian. Yet I bet even meat-lovers will tuck in. I love this as a Christmas dinner alternative or addition, as the flavours of Stilton always make me feel festive. If you want a vegan recipe, you can omit the Stilton, use vegan gluten-free puff pastry and brush with dairy-free milk instead of egg.

700g frozen chopped butternut squash
1 tbsp fresh sage leaves, chopped
2 tsp chopped garlic
1 red onion, chopped
Pinch of sea salt
2 tbsp olive oil
100g Stilton cheese
Gluten-free plain flour, for dusting

2 quantities chilled Rough Puff Pastry (see page 40)
1 egg, beaten

For the mushrooms
250g chestnut mushrooms
2 tsp chopped garlic
1 tsp dried thyme
1 tbsp olive oil
½ red onion, chopped
1 tbsp tamari sauce

Serves 6-8

1 Preheat the oven to 200ºC/Fan 180ºC/Gas Mark 6.

2 Place the squash in a large roasting tray along with the sage, garlic, onion and sea salt. Drizzle with the olive oil and mix well. Roast for 30 minutes, then set aside to cool completely.

3 While the squash is cooking, slice the mushrooms and add to a frying pan along with the garlic, thyme, olive oil, onion and tamari. Place over a medium heat and fry for 5–6 minutes, until the mushrooms have softened.

4 Blitz the mushroom mixture in a food processor, then allow to cool completely.

5 When everything has cooled, crumble the Stilton into the squash tray and mix well, until evenly distributed.

6 When you're ready to construct the Wellington, preheat the oven to 220ºC/Fan 200ºC/Gas Mark 7.

7 Lightly flour a work surface and roll out the chilled pastry so it is 4–5mm thick. Cut into 2 equal rectangles about 30 x 20cm.

8 Place a pastry rectangle on a sheet of baking paper and spread the mushroom mixture over it, leaving a clear 5cm border around the sides.

9 Spoon the squash mixture evenly over the mushrooms.

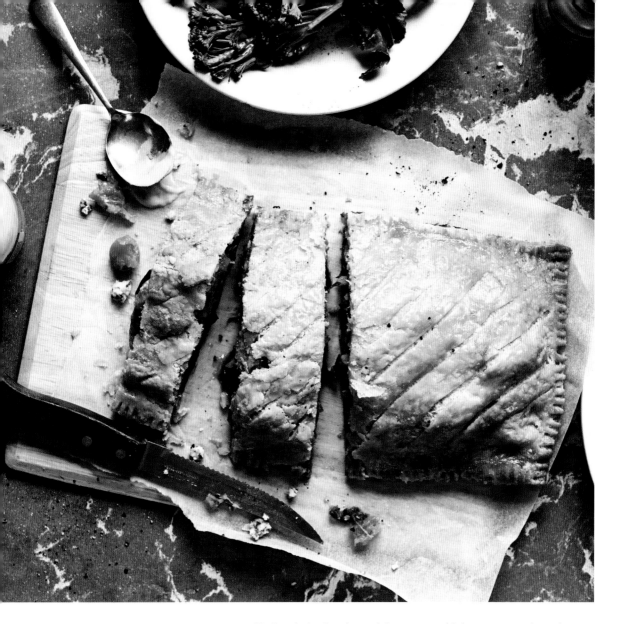

10 Brush the borders of the pastry with beaten egg, then place the remaining sheet of pastry on top and press the edges together. Trim off any excess with a sharp knife, then use a fork to firmly press the edges together. If you like, cut decorative shapes from the trimmings (without rerolling) and use a little beaten egg to stick them to the Wellington.

11 Place the Wellington on a baking tray and brush all over with beaten egg. Use a fork or the tip of a knife to make a few steam holes.

12 Bake for 25–30 minutes, until golden brown. Remove from the oven and leave to rest for 5 minutes before slicing and serving with roast potatoes and your choice of vegetables, plus some gluten-free gravy if you fancy it.

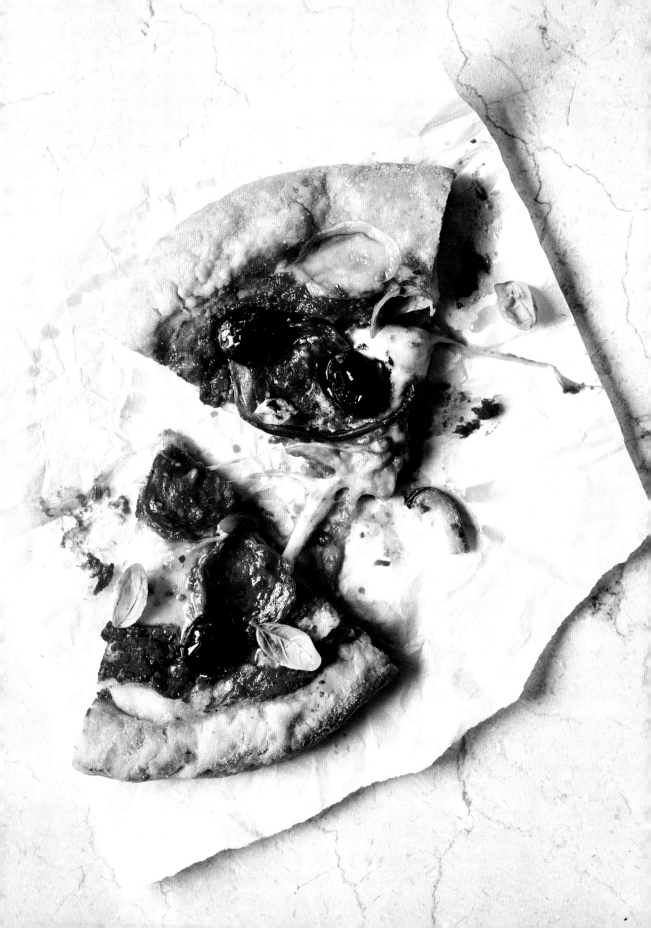

FAKEAWAY TREATS

Hands up those who skipped straight to this chapter because they're fed up with missing out on their favourite takeaways? Well, the alternatives in the following pages will have gluten-eaters drooling over your food. From the Chinese dishes I wish I could scoff, to proper-sized pizzas, authentic-tasting kebabs and the 'best of beige' – aka anything battered or breaded – I've got GF treats here for all meals and occasions.

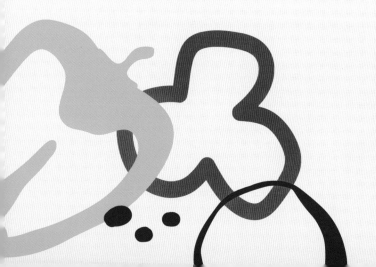

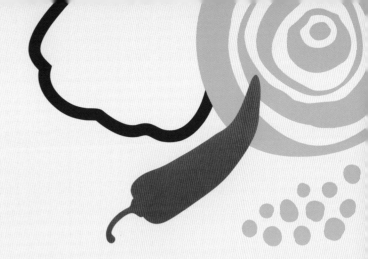

THE RECIPES

Chow Mein

Prep: **5 minutes**
Cook: **10 minutes**

DF

What you see is what you get with this dish, as chow mein means literally 'stir-fried noodles'. Traditional chow mein recipes use shaoxing rice wine, which contains gluten, so I always turn to good ol' sherry instead. It adds the same kick, and a bonus is that you can also use it to make a trifle. A win all round.

1 quantity Egg Noodles (see page 42), or 1 x 300g packet rice noodles
Toasted sesame oil, for coating and frying
200g chopped chicken breast
1 tsp chopped garlic
1 tsp chopped ginger
200g fresh mixed stir-fry vegetables
50g beansprouts
4 spring onions, chopped
Salt and pepper

For the sauce
3 tbsp tamari sauce
4 tsp dry sherry
1 tbsp cornflour
2 tbsp toasted sesame oil
1 tsp chopped ginger
1 tsp caster sugar

Serves 4

1 Start by making the sauce. Place the tamari, sherry and cornflour in a bowl and stir well until smooth. Add the sesame oil, ginger and sugar, stir again, then set to one side.

2 To cook the egg noodles, add them to a large pan of vigorously boiling salted water. Bring back to the boil and simmer for about 2 minutes, stirring occasionally to ensure they don't stick. If using ready-made rice noodles, cook them as per the packet instructions. Drain, transfer to a bowl and toss them in a little toasted sesame oil to stop them from sticking together.

3 Place a little more toasted sesame oil in a wok or large frying pan over a high heat. Once hot, add the chicken, garlic and ginger plus some salt and pepper. Stir-fry for 3–4 minutes, until brown.

4 Add the stir-fry veg, beansprouts and three-quarters of the spring onions. Stir-fry for another 2–3 minutes.

5 Add the cooked noodles to the pan and mix well.

6 Give the sauce a good stir in case the cornflour has settled at the bottom, then pour it over the noodles. Stir-fry for another minute, ensuring everything is well coated. Serve straight away, garnished with the remaining spring onions.

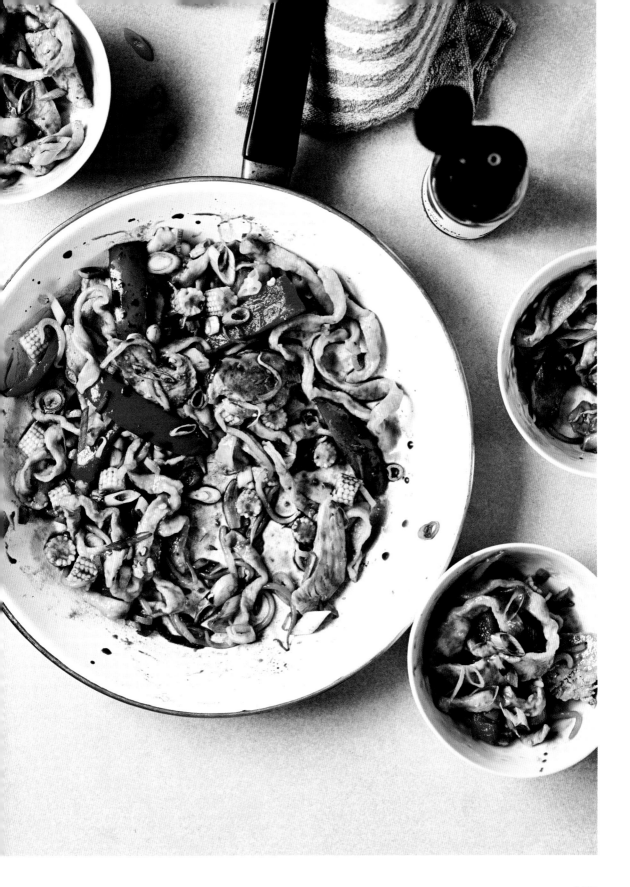

Singapore Noodles

Prep: **5 minutes**
Cook: **5 minutes**

DF

1 tbsp curry powder
1 tsp ground turmeric
1 tbsp tamari sauce
2 tsp chopped garlic
2 tbsp water
2 tbsp toasted sesame oil
100g raw frozen king prawns
100g cooked ham, chopped into small pieces
100g beansprouts
1 red pepper, deseeded and finely sliced
3 spring onions, chopped
1 quantity Egg Noodles (see page 42)

You often come across this dish made with rice noodles, but, as I've missed out on egg noodles for so long, I'm mixing things up a little here. Not only do chewy gluten-free egg noodles work really well in this dish, I also find them more satisfying.

Serves 4

1 Bring a large pan of salted water to the boil.

2 Meanwhile, place the curry powder, turmeric, tamari, chopped garlic and water in a small bowl and mix well. Stir in 1 tablespoon of the toasted sesame oil and set aside.

3 Place the remaining sesame oil in a wok or large frying pan over a high heat. Once hot, add the prawns and stir-fry for 1–2 minutes, until they are completely pink.

4 Add the chopped ham, beansprouts, red pepper and all but a handful of the spring onions. Stir-fry for 2–3 minutes.

5 When the water is boiling, add the noodles and simmer for 2 minutes, stirring occasionally to ensure they don't stick. Meanwhile, add the sauce mixture to the wok and stir well.

6 Drain the noodles and add them to the wok, using tongs to mix them thoroughly with the meat, veg and sauce. Serve straight away with the remaining spring onion sprinkled on top.

TOP TIP

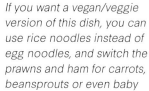

If you want a vegan/veggie version of this dish, you can use rice noodles instead of egg noodles, and switch the prawns and ham for carrots, beansprouts or even baby corn.

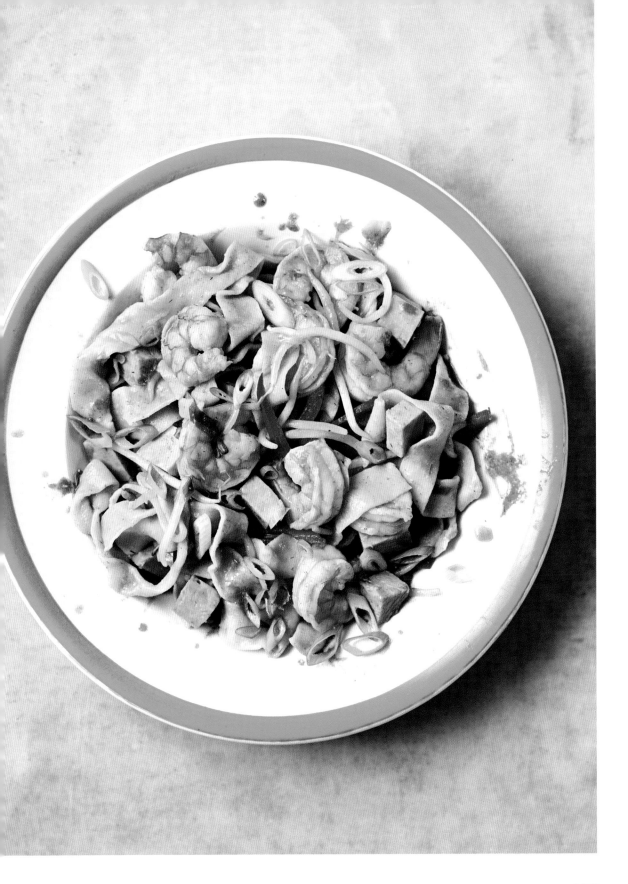

Soy, Chilli & Garlic Noodles

4 tbsp tamari sauce
2 tsp cornflour
1 quantity Egg Noodles
(see page 42)

2 tbsp toasted sesame oil, plus
extra for the noodles
6 tsp chopped garlic
1 red chilli, finely chopped
6 spring onions, finely chopped

Prep: **5 minutes**
Cook: **5 minutes**

 DF MF

It doesn't get much quicker than this when it comes to an easy fakeaway meal, especially if you've already made the egg noodles in advance. This is exactly the bowl of spicy, umami goodness I craved for so many years after my coeliac diagnosis. You can add any veg of your choosing – or even chicken or prawns – but I like to keep it simple for an easy bowl of yumminess.

Serves 4

1 Place the tamari and cornflour in a bowl and mix until smooth.

2 Add the egg noodles to a large pan of vigorously boiling salted water. Bring back to the boil and simmer for about 2 minutes, stirring occasionally to ensure they don't stick. Drain, transfer to a bowl and toss them in a little toasted sesame oil to stop them from sticking together.

3 Place 1 tablespoon of the sesame oil in a wok or large frying pan over a high heat. Once hot, add the garlic, chilli and spring onions and stir-fry for 1–2 minutes.

4 Add the cooked noodles to the pan, drizzle over another tablespoon of sesame oil and mix well. Stir in the tamari mixture and serve straight away.

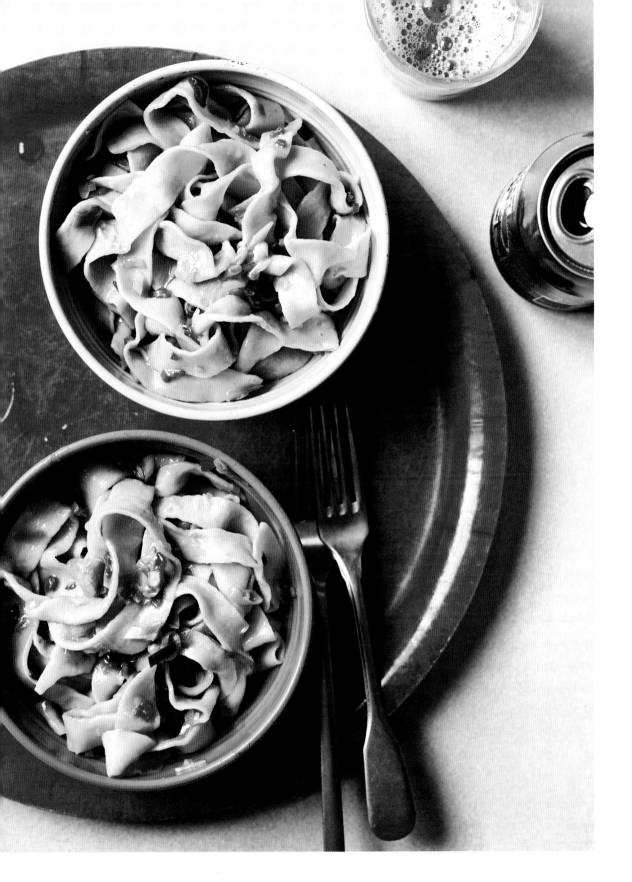

Salt & Pepper Squid

Prep: **5 minutes**
Cook: **10 minutes**

EF **DF**

Whether you have it as a starter or side, this crisp and delicious squid dish is one of my fakeaway favourites. It's surprisingly quick and easy to make and great served with egg fried rice or alongside another dish, such as my Sweet & Sour Pork (see page 188).

300g squid rings, defrosted if frozen
3 tbsp cornflour
1 tsp sea salt flakes
1 tsp ground black pepper
1 tsp Chinese five-spice powder
1 onion, chopped into 1–2cm chunks
3 spring onions, roughly chopped
2 tsp chopped garlic
1 red chilli, chopped into 1cm chunks
Vegetable oil, for frying

To serve
Lime wedges
Sweet chilli sauce, for dipping

Serves 4

1 Drain the squid rings and pat dry with kitchen paper.

2 Place the cornflour, salt, pepper and five-spice powder in a bowl and mix well. Add the squid rings and toss to coat thoroughly.

3 Pour a 1cm depth of oil into a wok or large frying pan and place over a high heat until it reaches 170ºC. (If you don't have a food thermometer, you can tell if the oil is hot enough when you dip in a wooden chopstick or the handle of a wooden spoon and little bubbles form around it.)

4 Add the squid rings to the hot oil a few at a time, ensuring they don't stick together. Fry for about 5 minutes, turning halfway through, until the coating is crispy.

5 Add the chopped onion, spring onions, garlic and chilli to the pan and stir-fry for another minute. Using a slotted spoon, transfer the squid and veg to a plate lined with kitchen paper to absorb any excess oil. Serve straight away with the lime wedges and sweet chilli sauce.

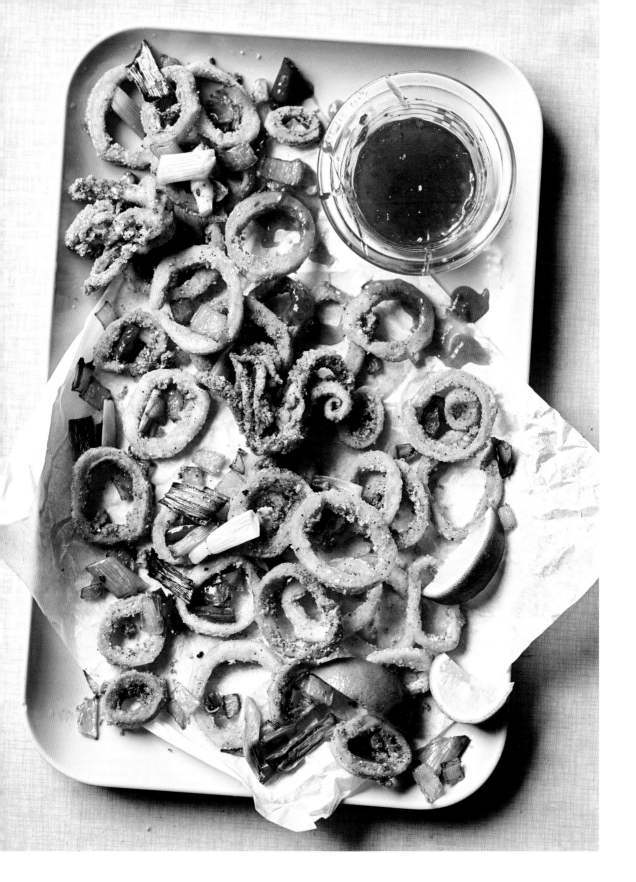

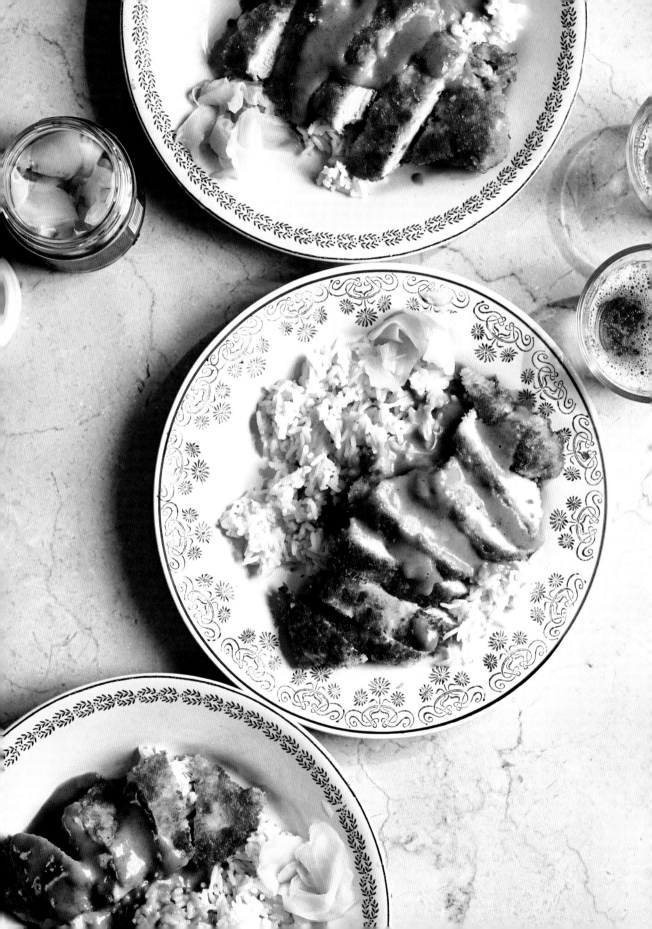

Katsu Curry

Prep: **5 minutes**
Cook: **30 minutes**

DF

Katsu curry is a perfect combination of crunchy breadcrumbed chicken and a creamy curry sauce. Making foods like this, which are so hard to get gluten free in a restaurant, is such a pleasure. The sheer delight of sitting in my PJs and crunching into that GF fried chicken slathered in curry sauce gives me far more joy than sharing a table with strangers in a crammed restaurant.

2 skinless chicken breasts
2 tbsp gluten-free plain flour
2 large eggs
100g gluten-free panko bread-
    crumbs (see page 38)
2–3 tbsp vegetable oil, for frying
Salt and pepper
2 x 250g pouches microwave
    jasmine rice, to serve

For the curry sauce
1 tbsp vegetable oil
1 onion, finely chopped
2 carrots, cut into small chunks
3 tsp chopped garlic
2 tbsp gluten-free plain flour
1 tbsp mild curry powder
1 tsp garam masala
½ gluten-free chicken stock
    cube dissolved in 400ml
    boiling water
200ml coconut milk
1 tbsp tamari sauce
1 bay leaf
1 tbsp honey

Serves 4

1   Start by making the sauce. Heat the oil in a large pan and fry the onion, carrot and garlic over a low–medium heat for 6–8 minutes, until they start to soften.

2   Add the flour, curry powder and garam masala, mix well and cook for 30 seconds.

3   Gradually add the stock, stirring each addition until smooth.

4   Add the coconut milk, tamari, bay leaf and honey, stir well and bring to the boil. Lower the heat to a simmer and cook for 20 minutes, stirring regularly.

5   Meanwhile, cut the chicken breasts in half lengthways. Place the flour, eggs and panko on separate plates, seasoning the first with salt and pepper and lightly whisking the second.

6   Coat each piece of chicken first in the flour, then the egg, and finally the panko, pressing the crumbs so they stick to the meat.

7   Place the oil in a frying pan over a medium–high heat. Once hot, add the breaded chicken breasts – you want them to sizzle nicely as they go in. Cook for 5 minutes on each side, until golden.

8   Once the sauce has finished simmering, use a hand blender to blitz it until smooth. Take care, as it can splash.

9   To serve, microwave the rice and divide between 4 plates. Slice the chicken and place on the rice with the curry sauce poured on top.

Pizza Margherita

Prep: **1 hour 10 minutes**
Cook: **15 minutes**

If there's one thing in life I believe passionately, it's that nobody on a gluten-free diet should be deprived of good pizza. Oh, and that every pizza should be at least 30cm in diameter. Okay, that was two things – but the long and short of it is, why settle for rubbish gluten-free pizza from the shops when you can make the best pizza recipe in the world? For the best results, you'll want to make the dough fresh each time. I also recommend using a pizza mesh for baking purposes – they're cheap to buy – but a baking sheet can be used instead.

TOP TIP

Pizza Margherita is the basic type that most others derive from. If you're feeling fancy, you can add extra toppings, such as ham, pepperoni, olives, anchovies, veggie pieces – whatever you like!

400ml milk or dairy-free alternative
3 tsp sugar
14g dried yeast
500g gluten-free white bread flour, plus extra for dusting
2 tsp xanthan gum
1 tsp salt
4 tbsp olive oil

For the tomato sauce
1 tbsp olive oil
1 tsp dried basil
1 tsp dried oregano
1 tsp chopped garlic
250g tomato passata
2 tbsp tomato purée
Salt and pepper

For the topping
1 x 250g ball of mozzarella cheese or dairy-free alternative, torn into pieces
Fresh basil leaves

Makes 2 x 30cm pizzas ─────────

1 Measure the milk into a heatproof jug and place in the microwave on full power, heating it in 30-second blasts until its temperature hits about 40ºC. This should feel like skin temperature if you dip your finger in, but I recommend using a food thermometer to avoid any errors.

2 Stir the sugar into the warm milk until dissolved, then add the yeast and stir again. Cover with a tea towel and leave in a warm spot for 5–10 minutes to activate the yeast. When ready, it should have a lovely froth on top.

3 Place the flour, xanthan gum and salt in a large bowl and stir well. Pour in the frothy milk and beat with a wooden spoon until the mixture becomes claggy. At this point, beat in the olive oil until you have a smooth, slightly sticky dough that comes away from the side of the bowl. This step is an excellent arm workout!

4 Cover the bowl with a piece of oiled clingfilm and place in a warm spot for 40–60 minutes, until the dough is puffy and doubled in size.

5 Meanwhile, make the sauce. Place the olive oil in a frying pan over a low heat. Add the basil, oregano and garlic and fry for 1–2 minutes, stirring occasionally, until the garlic softens. Pour in the passata and tomato purée, and season with salt and pepper. Mix well, then simmer for 5 minutes. Remove from the heat.

6 Once the dough has proved, preheat the oven to 240ºC/Fan 220ºC/Gas Mark 9 (a good hot oven is essential). Also set out 2 pizza meshes or 2 non-stick baking sheets.

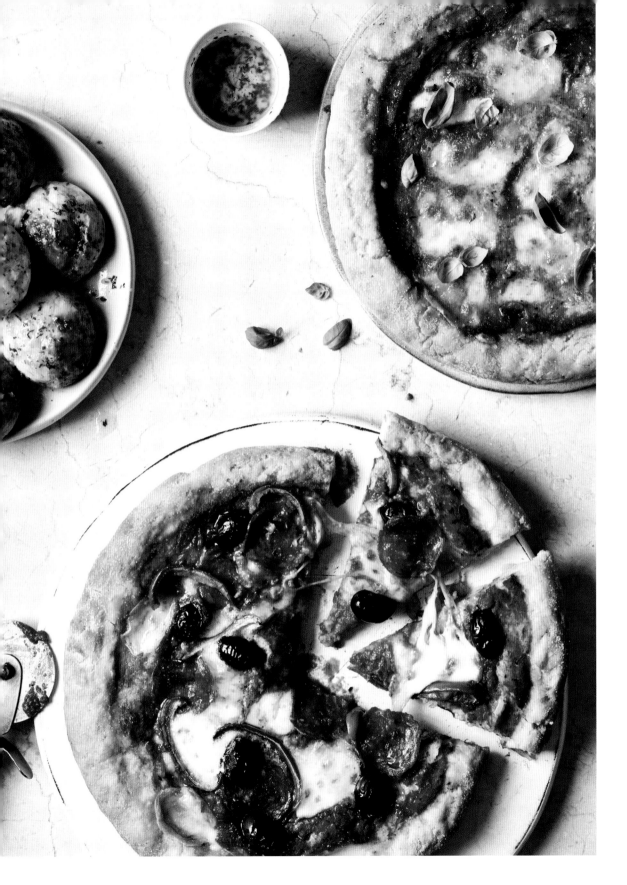

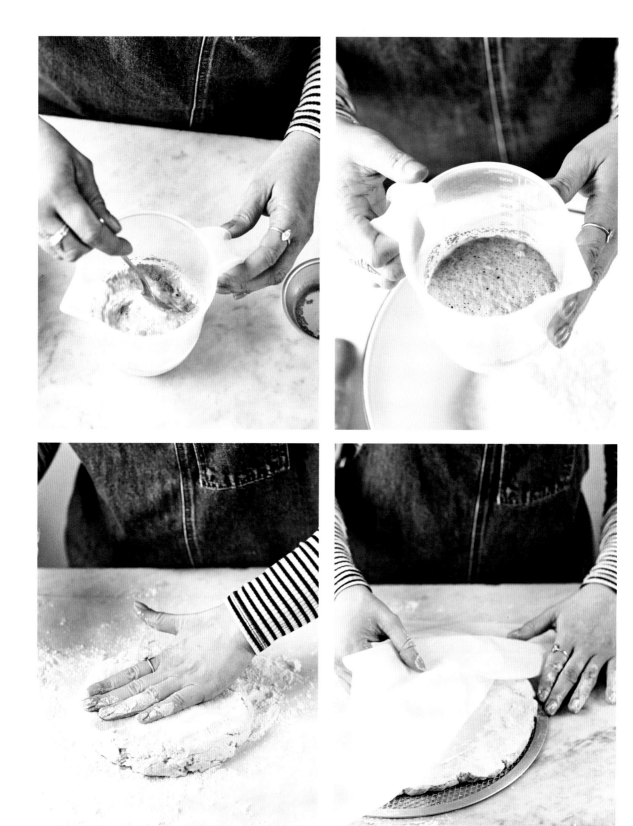

FAKEAWAY TREATS

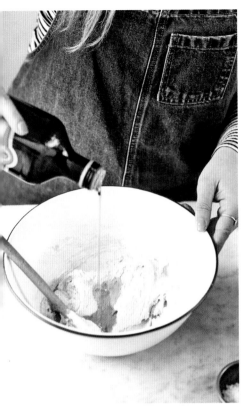

7 Place a 35cm length of baking paper on your work surface and dust it with a little extra flour. If you want to make a precise pizza shape, you can draw around a dinner plate on the paper to use as a guide, or just freestyle it.

8 Dust your hands with flour so the dough doesn't stick to them, then place half of it on the paper and gently push into a circular shape about 1–2cm thick and 30cm across.

9 Place a pizza mesh (if you have one) over the dough, then carefully lift the baking paper and flip it over so that the dough is sitting on the mesh. Alternatively, invert the pizza base onto a baking sheet. Carefully peel off the baking paper. Repeat this step to make a second pizza base.

10 Spread some of the tomato sauce over the pizza bases and dot with the mozzarella. Bake for 10–12 minutes, until the crust is golden brown and the cheese is bubbling. Sprinkle with the basil leaves and serve straight away with some Cheesy Dough Balls (see page 214).

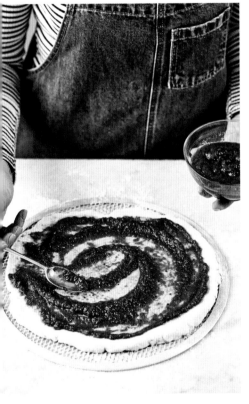

Stuffed-Crust Pizza

Prep: **1¼ hours**
Cook: **15 minutes**

Take my gluten-free pizza recipe (on page 180) to the next level by making it with a stuffed crust. I don't know why you can't buy this type of GF pizza from takeaways and restaurants when they're not really that difficult to make. If you've got kids, they'll love getting hands on and rolling up the cheesy crust, ready to bake.

1 quantity pizza dough
  (see page 180)
1 quantity tomato sauce
  (see page 180)
Gluten-free white bread flour,
  for dusting
1 x 400g block of firm mozzarella

cheese, for the crust
1 x 250g ball of mozzarella
  cheese, for the topping
Selection of ham, pepperoni,
  olives, anchovies, etc.
Olive oil, for brushing the crust

Makes 2 x 25cm pizzas

1 Once the dough has proved, preheat the oven to 240ºC/Fan 220ºC/Gas Mark 9 (a good hot oven is essential). Also set out 2 pizza meshes or 2 non-stick baking sheets.

2 Place a 35cm length of baking paper on your work surface and dust it with a little extra flour. If you want to make a precise pizza shape, you can draw around a dinner plate on the paper to use as a guide, or just freestyle it.

3 Dust your hands with flour so that the dough doesn't stick to them, then place half of it on the paper and gently push into a circular shape about 1–2cm thick and 30cm across. This width includes a 5cm allowance for the stuffed crust.

4 Place a pizza mesh over the dough, then carefully lift the baking paper and flip it over so that the dough is sitting on the mesh. Alternatively, invert the pizza base onto a baking sheet. Carefully peel off the baking paper. Repeat this step to make a second pizza base.

5 Use your thumb to press right around the pizza, forming a circular 'ditch' about 2.5cm away from the edge.

6 Cut strips of the firm mozzarella about 1cm thick and lay them end-to-end in the ditch, until you have completed the circle.

7 Use a pastry brush and water to wet the dough beside the inner edge of the cheese, then fold the outer dough over it. Wet your hands and use your thumb and fingers to gently pinch the dough together to seal in the cheese. The dough can be quite fragile, so take your time and use the wetness to pinch together any breaks that might occur. Keeping your fingers wet will stop the dough sticking to you, and dabbing a little extra flour onto the wet dough can also help to seal any cracks.

8 Spread half the tomato sauce over the pizza base, stopping about 1cm away from the stuffed crust.

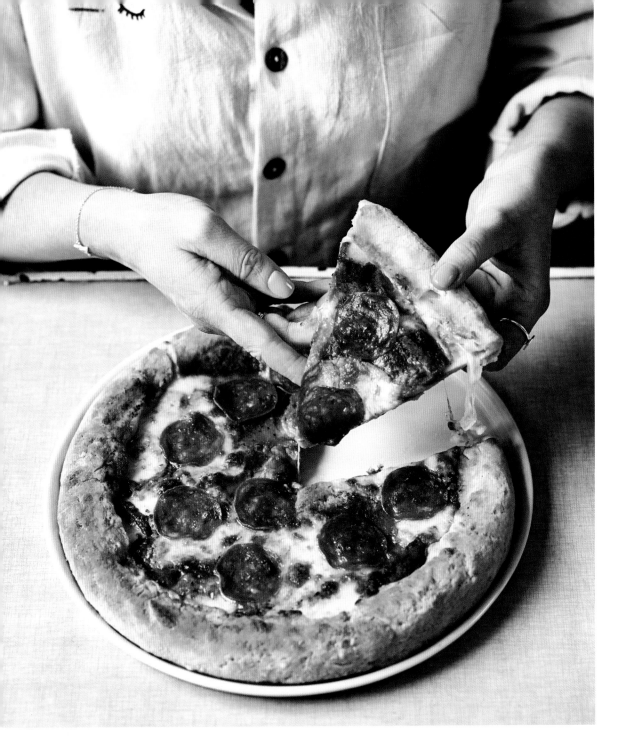

9 Tear the ball of mozzarella into pieces and dot over the sauce along with your chosen toppings. Brush around the crust with a little olive oil.

10 Carefully place the pizza in the oven and bake for 10–12 minutes, until the crust is golden brown and the top is bubbling. Slice up and serve hot.

Fantastic Fried Chicken

Prep: **10 minutes**
(+ overnight marinating)

Cook: **20 minutes**

EF

Fried chicken is my guilty pleasure, and this GF version (aka FFC) is the perfect takeaway dupe. Marinating the meat overnight in buttermilk makes it super-juicy and tender, while the golden, lightly spiced coating has the perfect crunch. KF-Who?

650g skinless chicken thigh fillets
200ml buttermilk
1.5 litres vegetable oil

For the coating
200g gluten-free plain flour
100g cornflour
2 tsp baking powder

2 tsp smoked paprika
2 tsp dried oregano
2 tsp cayenne pepper
1 tsp onion salt
1 tsp garlic granules
1 tsp dried thyme
1 tsp dried marjoram
½ tsp ground black pepper

Serves 4

1 Trim any excess fat from the chicken fillets and open them out flat. Place in a large container or dish, add the buttermilk and mix well. Cover and leave to marinate in the fridge for up to 24 hours, but at least 8.

2 Place all the coating ingredients in a large tub, cover with a lid and shake well.

3 When you're ready to fry the chicken, place the oil in a large, deep pan and heat to 170°C. (If you don't have a food thermometer, you can tell if the oil is hot enough when you dip in a wooden chopstick or the handle of a wooden spoon and little bubbles form around it.)

4 Stir the chicken to make sure it's well coated in the buttermilk. Place one piece at a time in the coating, pressing down on both sides to ensure it's evenly covered. Repeat this step with all the chicken pieces.

5 Using tongs, carefully lower the coated chicken, one piece at a time, into the oil, frying no more than 2–3 bits together. You want to make sure the chicken is completely submerged and that the pieces don't touch, so don't try to cram them all in at once. Fry for 4 minutes, ensuring the temperature of the oil stays around 170°C.

6 Using tongs, transfer the chicken to a plate lined with kitchen paper. If you want to check the chicken is cooked through, cut into the thickest part to ensure it's not pink, or insert a food thermometer, which should register at least 75°C.

7 Cook all the chicken pieces in the same way, then serve hot with chips, salad or in gluten-free burger buns or wraps.

TOP TIP

To turn this dish into popcorn chicken, simply cut the chicken thigh fillets into 5–7.5cm chunks before marinating in the buttermilk. Toss them in the coating and fry for 2–3 minutes. As you see, there's no actual popcorn involved; the fried chunks just become crispy, like popcorn.

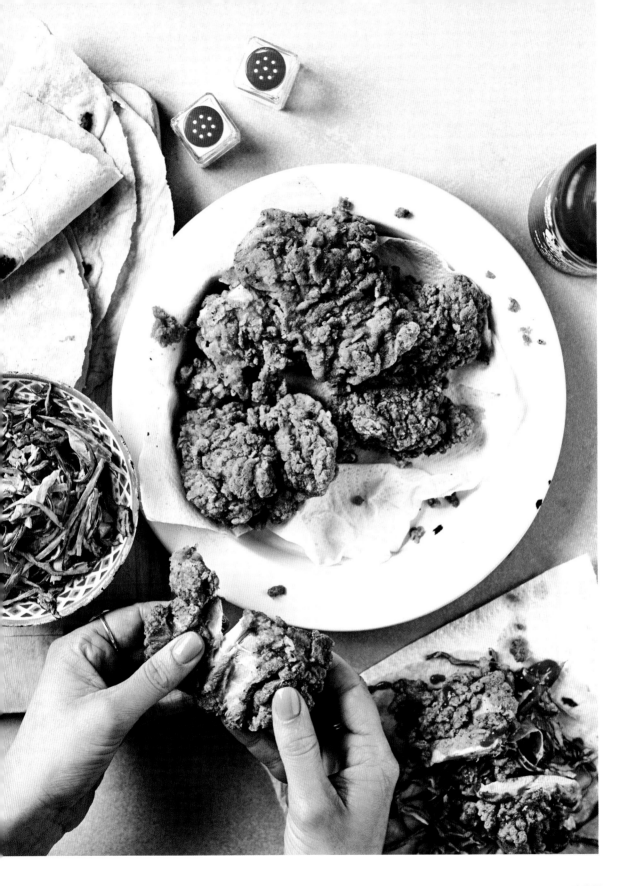

Sweet & Sour Pork

Prep: **20 minutes**
(+ up to 48 hours marinating)

Cook: **25 minutes**

EF   **DF**

600g pork shoulder, cut into
  5cm chunks
About 1 litre vegetable oil
65g cornflour
1 red pepper, deseeded and cut
  into chunks
1 yellow pepper, deseeded and
  cut into chunks
1 large onion, cut into chunks
1 x 220g tin pineapple chunks,
  drained and juice reserved

For the marinade
2 tbsp tamari sauce
1 tsp garlic granules

1 tsp ginger purée
½ tsp baking powder
2 tsp cornflour

For the sauce
130g tomato ketchup
2 tbsp tamari sauce
4 tbsp caster sugar
4 tbsp white rice vinegar or
  apple cider vinegar
2 tsp chopped garlic
200ml reserved pineapple juice
2 tbsp cornflour mixed with 4
  tbsp cold water

If there was one takeaway dish that really made my seething snakes of envy emerge, it was sweet and sour pork. That's why I genuinely shed a tear when I finally created a successful GF version of this classic. Trust me on the pork shoulder – I know it's more commonly used for slow cooking, but the marinade helps to break down the fibres, so it becomes super-tender. If you can leave it to marinate for a full 48 hours, it's worth it.

Serves 4

1   Combine the marinade ingredients in a large tub. Add the pork and mix well to coat. Cover and marinate in the fridge for up to 48 hours, but at least 12, stirring occasionally.

2   When you're ready to cook, heat the oven to its lowest setting. Pour a 2.5cm depth of the oil into a large saucepan and heat to about 170ºC. (If you don't have a food thermometer, you can tell if the oil is hot enough when you dip in a wooden chopstick or the handle of a wooden spoon and little bubbles form around it.)

3   Tip the marinated pork into a large bowl and stir in the cornflour until the meat is completely coated. Using tongs, add 6–10 pieces of pork one at a time to the hot oil. The number depends on how big your pan is, as you want the cubes to have some space. Fry for 5 minutes, then use a slotted spoon to transfer the pieces to an ovenproof dish. Keep warm in the oven while you fry the remaining pork in similar sized batches. Once all the pork is cooked, combine the sauce ingredients in a bowl or jug and mix well.

4   Place 1–2 teaspoons vegetable oil in a wok over a high heat. When hot, add the peppers and onions and stir-fry for 2–3 minutes, until they start to brown but are still crunchy.

5   Lower the heat to medium, pour in the sauce mixture and cook, stirring, for 2–3 minutes, until it has thickened and become more vibrant in colour.

6   Add the fried pork and pineapple chunks to the sauce, stir to coat and serve straight away with Egg Fried Rice (see page 208).

TOP TIP

This dish is definitely best eaten at the time of making. If you need to make it ahead, I recommend storing the cooked pork and sauce separately to retain the pork's crispness. Reheat the sauce in a large pan, then add the pork and cook for 5–6 minutes, until the pork is hot right through.

Chicken & Cashew Nuts

Prep: **5 minutes**
Cook: **10 minutes**

EF   DF

As this dish was a long-time favourite of mine from the Chinese takeaway, I vowed to create a GF version, and spent ages trying to get it bang on. The result is great, even if I do say so myself, and it's ready in just 15 minutes, so you can be eating while other people are still waiting for their food to be delivered.

2 tbsp vegetable oil
4 boneless, skinless chicken thigh fillets, sliced into 1cm strips
1 white onion, roughly chopped into chunks
3 garlic cloves, crushed
1 green pepper, deseeded and chopped into chunks

100g cashew nuts

For the sauce
3 tbsp tamari sauce
1 tbsp cornflour
1 tbsp toasted sesame oil
1 tsp white rice vinegar
160ml cold water

Serves 4

1   Combine all the sauce ingredients in a bowl and mix until smooth.

2   Place the oil in a wok or large frying pan over a high heat. Once hot, check the temperature with a small piece of chicken: the oil is hot enough if the test piece sizzles as soon as it hits the pan. At this point, add the chicken strips and stir-fry for 2–3 minutes, until they start to brown.

3   Add the onion, garlic and pepper, and continue to stir-fry for 2–3 minutes. You want the veg to stay relatively crunchy, so frying on a high heat for a short time is key here.

4   Pour in the sauce, mix well and cook, stirring, for 1–2 minutes, until it starts to thicken.

5   Stir in the cashew nuts and serve immediately with Egg Fried Rice (see page 208).

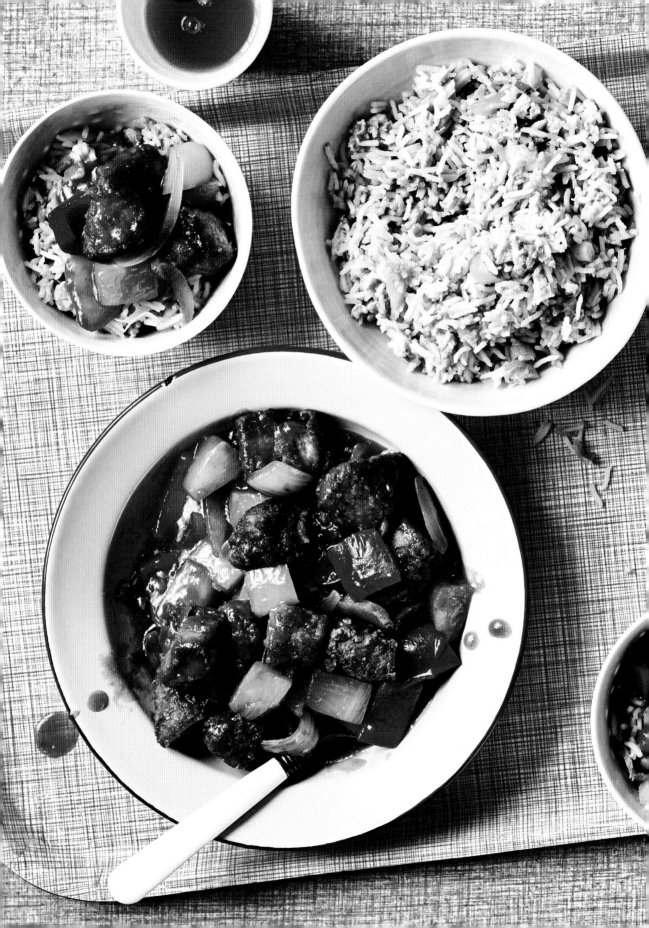

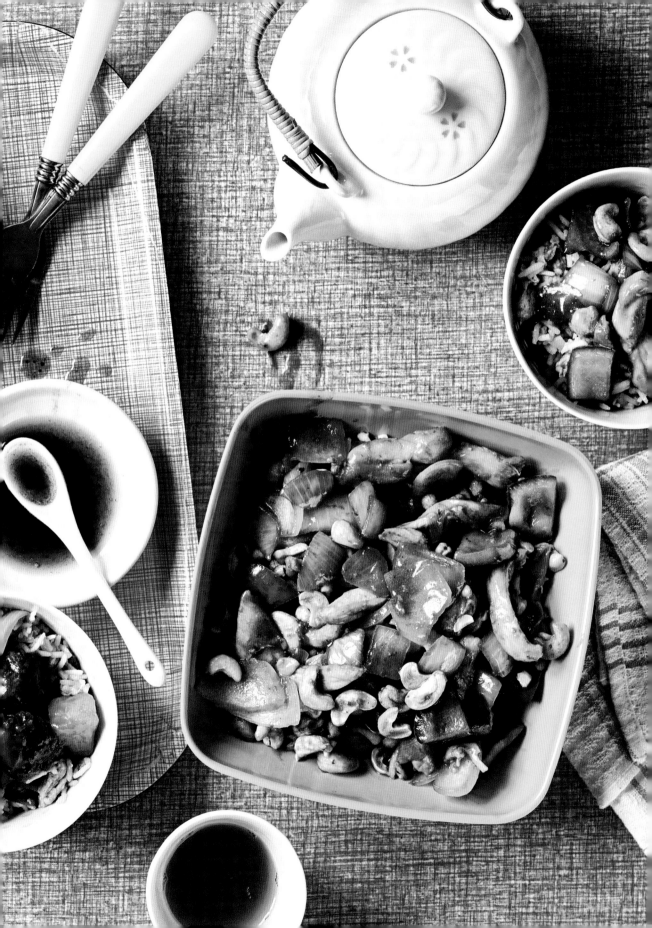

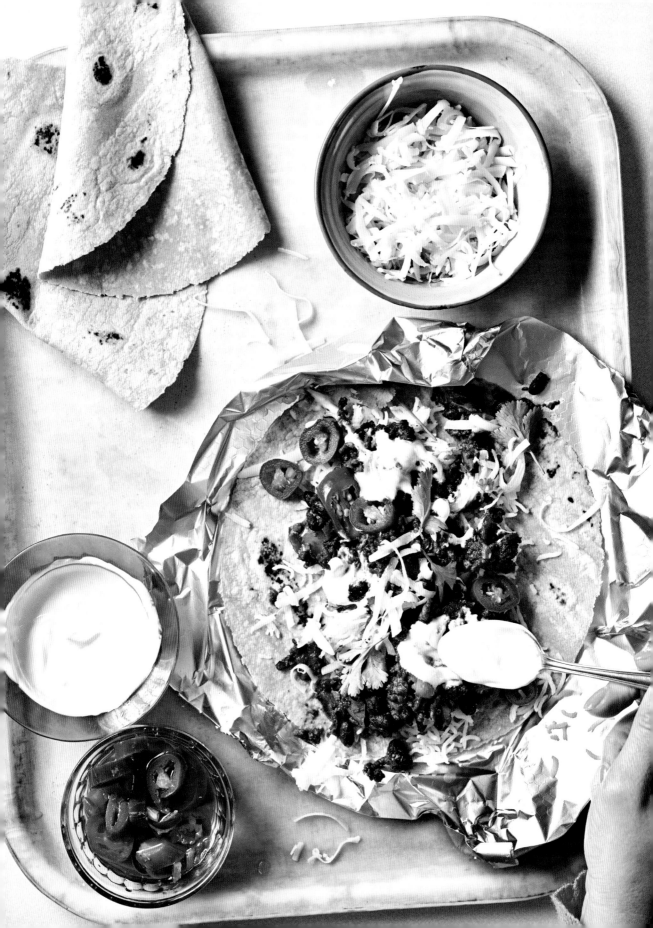

Brilliant Beef Burritos

Prep: **5 minutes**
Cook: **45 minutes**

When you need a grab-and-go idea for lunch or dinner, you just can't beat a beef burrito. A spicy beef chilli mingles with melty cheese, tender rice and fiery jalapeños, all wrapped up in a gluten-free tortilla blanket. Unwrap and eat straight from the foil casing to save on washing up.

1 tbsp olive oil
1 onion, finely chopped
2 tsp chopped garlic
1 yellow pepper, deseeded and chopped
1 green pepper, deseeded and chopped
500g lean beef mince
2 tsp mild chilli powder
2 tsp regular paprika
1 tsp smoked paprika
1 tsp ground cumin
1 tsp dried oregano
1 tsp cayenne pepper
1 tsp salt
1 x 400g tin chopped tomatoes
1 x 400g tin black beans, drained
1 x 10g square dark chocolate at least 70% cocoa solids)
8 gluten-free Tortilla Wraps (see page 37)
2 x 250g pouches microwave basmati rice
2–3 tbsp chopped jalapeños, from a jar (optional)
160g Cheddar cheese or dairy-free alternative, grated

Serves 4

1   Place the olive oil in a large frying pan over a medium heat. Once hot, add the onion, garlic and peppers and fry for 4–5 minutes.

2   Add the beef mince, breaking it up with a spatula and mixing with the veg. Fry for 6–8 minutes, until brown all over.

3   Add the oregano, all the spices and salt and stir well. Tip in the tomatoes and black beans, add the chocolate and mix again. Bring to the boil, then lower the heat to a simmer and cook, stirring occasionally, for 10–15 minutes, until the liquid has reduced.

4   Preheat the oven to 200°C/Fan 180°C /Gas Mark 6.

5   Lay a tortilla wrap on a square of foil that is slightly larger than it. Place one-eighth of the rice on it in a line down the centre, leaving a 2.5–5cm space down either side. Spoon one-eighth of the beef mixture on top of the rice, sprinkle with some jalapeños, if using, and a small amount of cheese.

6   Place the wrap so the filling runs from left to right in front of you. Fold the bottom of the wrap over the filling, then curve your fingers around it and pull back slightly to tuck it underneath. Fold in the sides of the tortilla, then roll up completely into a tight cylinder.

7   Wrap the foil tightly around the burrito and place on a baking tray. Repeat steps 5 and 6 to make 7 more burritos. At this stage, they can be frozen, ready to defrost and cook whenever you need them.

8   Place the tray of burritos in the oven for 15–20 minutes, then serve straight away.

TOP TIP

Don't like the filling so spicy? Try halving the cayenne pepper and chilli powder and serving the burritos with soured cream for dipping. Alternatively, to ramp up the heat, you can use hot chilli powder instead of mild.

Chicago-Style Deep-Pan Pizza

Prep: **1 hour 5 minutes**
Cook: **35 minutes**

The idea of a Chicago-style pizza – with the cheese under the sauce, and a thick-walled crust around it – has always intrigued me. I could never quite get my head around it, but now I've tried it, I'm completely converted. Polenta in the crust gives it a tasty 'bite' and the whole thing is amazingly cheesy (I recommend using pre-grated mozzarella to avoid any excess moisture). This is now one of my favourite pizza recipes.

TOP TIP

To make this recipe dairy-free or vegan, simply use a dairy-free milk when making the base, and dairy-free cheeses for the filling and topping.

400ml milk
2 tsp caster sugar
14g dried yeast
440g gluten-free white bread flour, plus extra for dusting
60g gluten-free fine polenta
2 tsp xanthan gum
1 tsp salt
4 tbsp olive oil, plus extra fo greasing

For the tomato sauce
1 tbsp olive oil
1 onion, finely diced
3 tsp chopped garlic
2 x 400g tins finely chopped tomatoes
2 tbsp tomato purée
1 tsp caster sugar
½ tsp salt
1 tsp dried oregano
1 tsp dried basil

For the topping
1 x 250g mozzarella cheese, grated
70g pepperoni slices
20g Parmesan cheese, grated

Makes 2 x 20cm deep-pan pizzas _____

1   Measure the milk into a heatproof jug and place in the microwave on full power, heating it in 30-second blasts until it hits around 40ºC. This should feel like skin temperature if you dip your finger in, but I recommend using a food thermometer to avoid any errors.

2   Stir the sugar into the warm milk until dissolved, then add the yeast and stir again. Cover with a tea towel and leave in a warm spot for 5–10 minutes to activate the yeast. When ready, it should have a lovely froth on top.

3   Place the flour, polenta, xanthan gum and salt in a large bowl and stir well. Pour in the frothy milk and beat with a wooden spoon until the mixture becomes claggy. At this point, beat in the olive oil until you have a smooth, slightly sticky dough that comes away from the side of the bowl.

4   Cover the bowl with a piece of oiled clingfilm and place in a warm spot for 40–60 minutes, until the dough is puffy and doubled in size.

5   Meanwhile, make the sauce. Place the oil in a pan over a medium–low heat. Add the onion and garlic and fry for 6–8 minutes, until soft.

6   Add the tomatoes, tomato purée, sugar, salt and herbs and mix well. Bring to the boil, then lower the heat to a simmer and cook, uncovered, for 10–15 minutes, until the sauce has thickened.

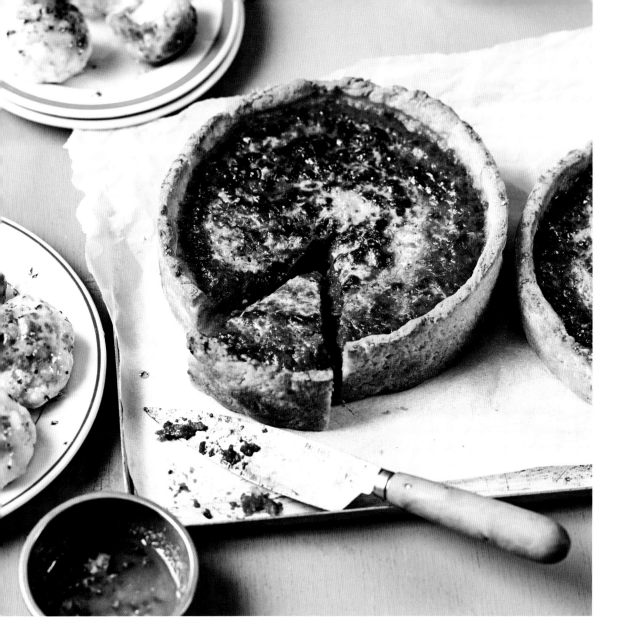

7 Once the dough has proved, preheat the oven to 240°C/Fan 220°C/Gas Mark 9 (a good hot oven is essential). Grease 2 x 20cm round cake tins with the extra olive oil.

8 Cut the dough in half, then wet your hands and roll each piece into a ball. Place a ball of dough in each tin and use wet hands to press it out, forming a flat base with a surrounding crust at least 2.5cm high.

9 Divide the mozzarella between the 2 pizza bases, spreading it evenly. Dot the pepperoni on top, then pour the sauce over so that it covers everything. Sprinkle with the Parmesan, then bake for 25–30 minutes, until the crust is golden and the filling is bubbling. Set aside for 5 minutes, before cutting up and serving hot.

Meatball Marinara Sub

Prep: **10 minutes**
Cook: **20 minutes**

'One 6-inch meatball sub, toasted with cheese, please!' These are the words I've always longed to say, but never been able to…until now! These homemade, meatball marinara submarine rolls are absolutely delicious, really quick to make, and just the best messy lunch. Definitely not first date food, but absolutely the way to a gluten-free person's heart.

250g lean beef mince
250 lean pork mince
40g gluten-free panko bread-crumbs
1 tbsp mixed Italian herbs
1 tsp salt
1 tsp onion salt
½ tsp garlic granules
1 large egg
1 tbsp olive oil

For the sauce
1 onion, finely chopped
2 tsp chopped garlic
1 tbsp olive oil
500ml tomato passata
2 tsp dried oregano
1 tsp dried basil
½ tsp dried thyme
½ tsp dried rosemary
¼ tsp chilli flakes

To serve
4 gluten-free sub-style rolls
8 slices mild Cheddar cheese or dairy-free alternative
4 tsp grated Parmesan cheese or dairy-free alternative

Serves 4

1 Make the meatballs by placing all the ingredients for them, except the oil, in a large bowl. Use your hands to 'squish' the mixture together until fully combined. Divide into 16 equal pieces, about 40g each, and roll into balls.

2 Place the oil in a frying pan over a medium heat. Once hot, add a batch of meatballs, well spaced out, and fry for 8–10 minutes, turning regularly until browned on all sides. Transfer to a plate lined with kitchen paper and set to one side. Cook the remaining meatballs in the same way.

3 To make the sauce, place the olive oil in a clean frying pan over a medium–low heat. Add the onion and garlic and fry for 3–4 minutes, until starting to soften. Pour in the passata, add the herbs and chilli flakes, and mix well.

4 Add the meatballs to the sauce, bring to the boil, then simmer for 5 minutes.

5 Preheat the oven to 180ºC/Fan 160ºC/Gas Mark 4.

6 Place the bread rolls on a baking tray and slit them open lengthways so they are still hinged together. Place 2 slices of the cheese in each roll, add 4 meatballs per roll and divide the sauce equally between them. Sprinkle with the Parmesan, then pop the baking tray in the oven for 5–10 minutes, until the cheese is bubbling and the edges of the rolls have toasted. Serve straight away.

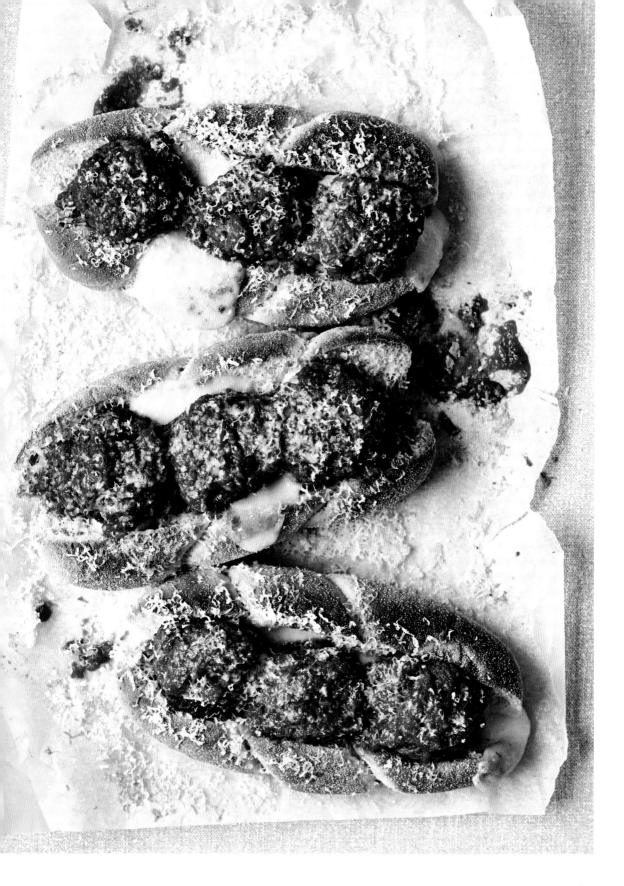

Beer-Battered Fish & Chips

Prep: **10 minutes**
(+ 20 minutes resting)

Cook: **35 minutes**

EF

Here's my version of a British takeaway classic – gorgeously crisp, golden and gluten-free. I prefer to make oven chips, which are slightly healthier than deep-fried ones, and conveniently ready by the time you've prepped and cooked the fish. The batter is made with gluten-free beer and puffs up beautifully, creating a crunchy coating for the flaky white cod. Serving this meal in newspaper is optional.

75g gluten-free plain flour, plus extra for sprinkling
50g cornflour
1 tsp baking powder
150ml gluten-free beer
Pinch of salt
4 skinless and boneless cod fillets (about 500g in total)
1 litre vegetable oil, for deep-frying

For the chips
1kg Maris Piper or King Edward potatoes, unpeeled
2 tbsp vegetable oil
Pinch of sea salt flakes

To serve
Gluten-free vinegar
Ketchup and/or Tartare Sauce (see page 72)

Serves 4

1 Place the plain flour, cornflour and baking powder in a large bowl and mix together. Gradually pour in the beer, whisking constantly, until you have a smooth, runny batter. Add a pinch of salt, whisk again and set aside to rest for at least 20 minutes.

2 Meanwhile, preheat the oven to 220ºC/Fan 200ºC/Gas Mark 7. Bring a large pan of water to the boil.

3 Cut the potatoes into chips about 2 cm thick. Add them to the pan of boiling water, bring back to the boil and cook, covered, for 2–3 minutes. Drain well, return them to the pan and add the 2 tablespoons vegetable oil and the salt flakes. Put the lid back on and toss them gently to coat.

4 Tip the chips into a roasting tray, spacing them evenly. Pop in the oven for 30 minutes, turning them over halfway through.

5 Meanwhile, pour a 7.5cm depth of vegetable oil into a large pan. Place over a high heat and bring it to 200ºC, checking the temperature with a food thermometer. Or test it by dropping in a small cube of bread, which should brown in 10 seconds.

6 When the oil has reached 200ºC, sprinkle the extra plain flour onto a plate. Dip one piece of cod in the flour, coating it well on both sides – this will help the batter to stick.

7 Give the batter a good stir, then dip the flour-coated cod in it. Lift out using tongs and carefully lower straight into the hot oil – don't drop it in or it will splash. Repeat with a second piece of fish if your pan is big enough to fit 2 pieces without touching, and cook for 4–5 minutes, until the batter is golden brown.

8 Carefully transfer the cooked fish to a plate lined with kitchen paper, and repeat the coating and cooking process with the remaining fish. Serve with the chips, salt and gluten-free vinegar, plus a good dollop of ketchup or tartare sauce.

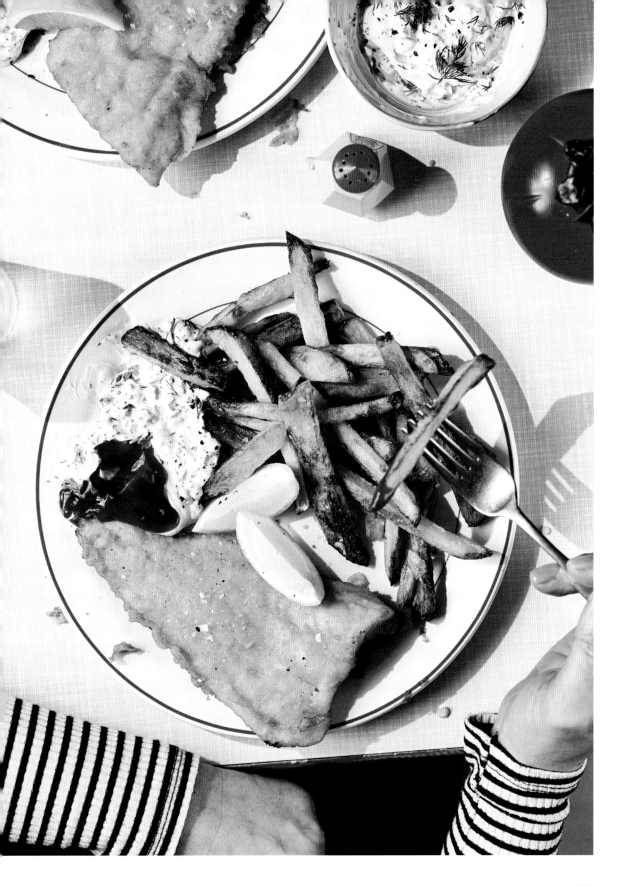

Doner Kebab

Prep: **10 minutes**
Cook: **50 minutes**

500g lamb mince or beef mince, at least 20% fat
1 tsp salt
½ tsp caster sugar
½ tsp bicarbonate of soda
1 tsp dried oregano
1 tsp ground cumin
1 tsp paprika
1 tsp mild chilli powder
½ tsp garlic granules
½ tsp onion salt
¼ tsp ground black pepper
¼ tsp ground cinnamon

For the garlic sauce

150g natural yoghurt or dairy-free alternative
3 tsp garlic paste
Juice of ½ lemon
1 tsp mint sauce

To serve

4 gluten-free pitta breads
Iceberg lettuce
1 red onion, finely sliced

I've always wanted to enjoy a greasy, delicious doner kebab, but usually they're made with breadcrumbs or gluten-containing spice mixes. This at-home, gluten-free version is surprisingly easy to make, and ideal for a delicious treat. A perfect kebab relies on fatty meats, so make sure you use at least 20% fat beef or lamb mince for optimum flavour. I recommend keeping some leftovers in the freezer for 2am hangover-prevention purposes.

Serves 4

1 Preheat the oven to 180ºC/Fan 160ºC/Gas Mark 4.

2 Place the mince in a large bowl. In a separate bowl, thoroughly combine the salt, sugar, bicarbonate of soda, oregano and all the spices. Add to the mince, mix with a wooden spoon, then use your hands to 'squish' everything together.

3 Shape the mince into a large, fat sausage about 18cm long. Place it in the centre of a large sheet of foil and wrap tightly so that no steam can escape during cooking. Place in a roasting tray and bake for 35–40 minutes, until the meat is completely cooked through. Set aside for 10 minutes.

4 Meanwhile, combine the garlic sauce ingredients in a bowl. Toast the pitta breads and shred the lettuce.

5 Preheat the grill until very hot.

6 Carefully unwrap the meat, reserving the foil and cooking juices, and transfer to a chopping board. Carve the meat into thin slices. Lay the cooking foil out in the roasting tray, keeping the juices in place, then spread the sliced meat on top. Grill for 1–2 minutes, until it browns. Serve in the pitta breads with shredded lettuce, some sliced onion and a good drizzle of garlic sauce.

TOP TIP

If you're feeding fewer than 4 people, you can always freeze the extra meat for another time. Simply slice it up and freeze before grilling, then defrost and reheat under the grill before serving. The sauce is best made fresh each time, but will keep in the fridge for 1–2 weeks.

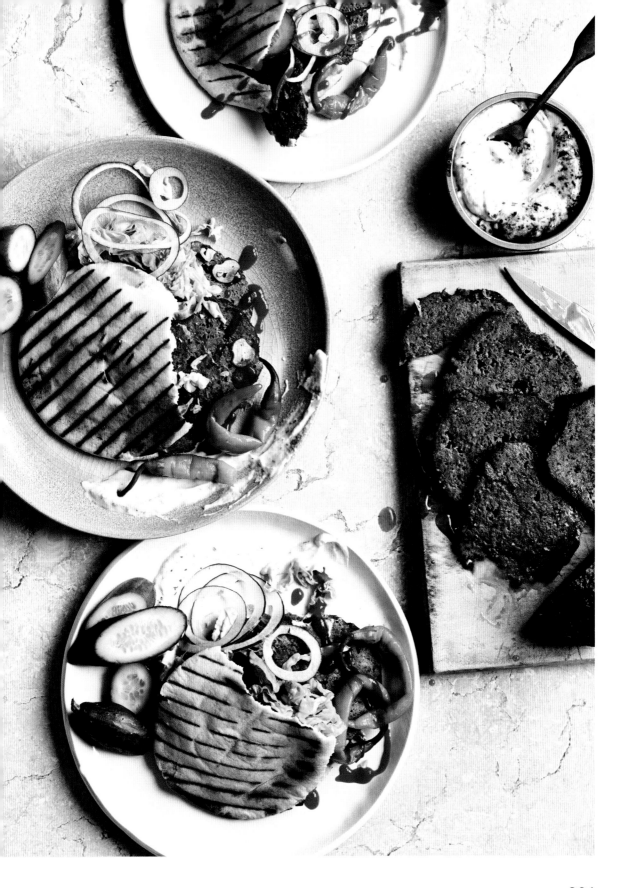

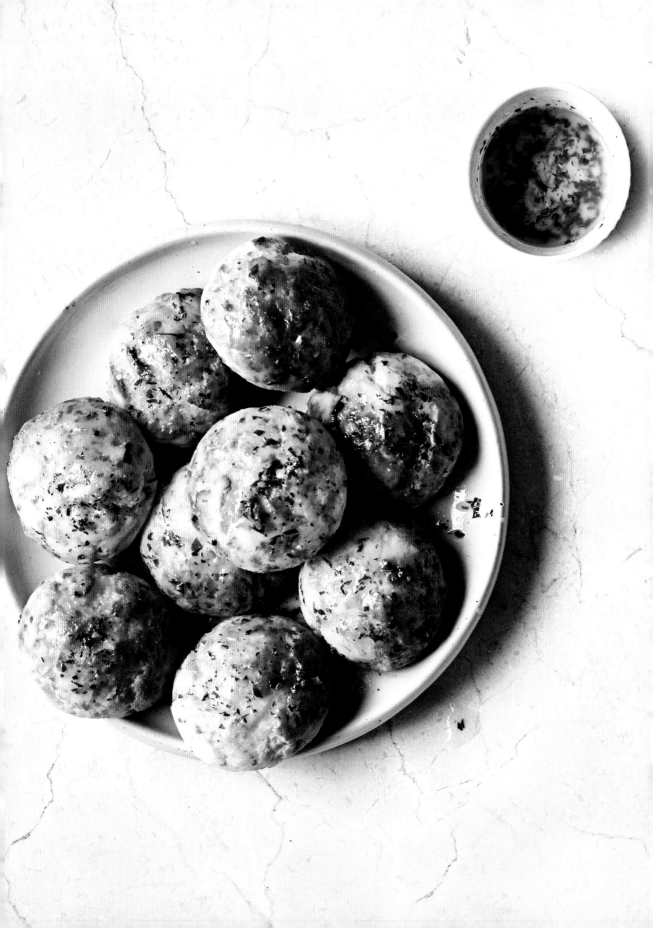

BITS ON THE SIDE

What delicious gluten-free meal would be complete without a selection of side dishes? This is so often the part of a meal we coeliacs miss out on, so in this chapter I've aimed to give you plenty of choice. From simple bread recipes to spring rolls, bhajis, Yorkshire puds and potatoes galore, you can find the perfect partner for any dish. Or, if you're anything like me, whip up a few of them in one go for a main course and call it 'Picky Bits'.

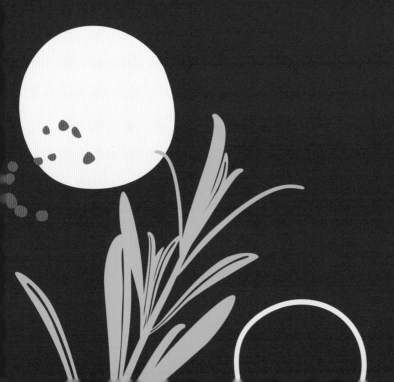

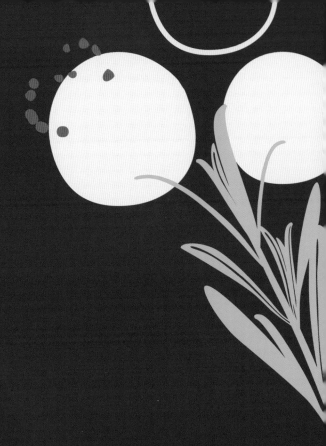

THE RECIPES

Sage & Onion Stuffing Balls

200g gluten-free white bread
1 tbsp vegetable oil
1 red onion, finely chopped
1 white onion, finely chopped
1 tbsp fresh sage, finely
  chopped

1 tsp dried sage
½ tsp onion salt
1 garlic clove, crushed
2 eggs, beaten

Prep: **10 minutes**
Cook: **40 minutes**

Sometimes shortcuts are a false economy, and cutting corners when making stuffing balls is a case in point. The secret to the awesome taste in my recipe is to toast the breadcrumbs first and to use double sage and double onion. Trust me, I've tried to dodge doing these things and the result just isn't as good.

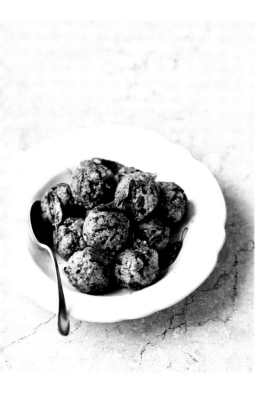

Makes 12

1 Preheat the oven to 220°C/Fan 200°C/Gas Mark 7. Line a baking tray with baking paper.

2 Blitz the bread in a food processor until it forms crumbs, then spread them out on a large baking tray. Bake for 10 minutes, using a spoon to stir them halfway through. Once golden, set aside to cool. Turn the oven down to 200°C/Fan 180°C/Gas Mark 6.

3 Place the oil in a large frying pan over a low heat. Once hot, fry the onions for 8–10 minutes, until they start to soften and brown.

4 Add the fresh sage, dried sage, onion salt and garlic. Stir and fry for 1 minute, then set aside to cool for 5 minutes.

5 Place the toasted breadcrumbs and onion mixture in a bowl, add the eggs and mix with a wooden spoon.

6 Wet your hands to prevent the mixture from sticking to them, then 'squish' the stuffing until it starts to clump together.

7 Break the mixture into 12 equal pieces and roll into balls. Space them out on the prepared tray.

8 Bake the stuffing balls for 25–30 minutes, until golden brown. Serve alongside your favourite roast dinner.

Yorkshire Puddings

12 tsp vegetable oil
75g gluten-free plain flour
75g cornflour

120ml milk
3 large eggs
Pinch of salt

Prep: **5 minutes**
Cook: **25 minutes**

Who can resist a Yorkshire pud?
So easy to make and the perfect
accompaniment to a Sunday roast or
Christmas dinner. The key to getting
them big and puffy is making sure
the oil is super-hot before you add
the batter. They also freeze well, and
reheat easily from frozen – simply pop
them in a hot oven for 5–10 minutes
before serving.

Makes 12

1   Preheat the oven to 220°C/Fan 200°C/Gas Mark 7.

2   Pour 1 teaspoon vegetable oil into each compartment
    of a 12-hole muffin tray and place in the oven for about
    10 minutes, until good and hot.

3   Meanwhile, make the batter. Place the flour and remaining
    ingredients in a large jug and whisk until smooth. Leave to sit
    at room temperature.

4   When the oil is hot, remove the tray from the oven. Working
    as quickly as possible, pour the batter into the 12 holes. It
    should roughly half-fill each hole and the oil should sizzle as
    the batter hits it.

5   Quickly return the tray to the oven and bake for
    18–20 minutes, until the puds are golden brown and
    puffed up. Serve straight away.

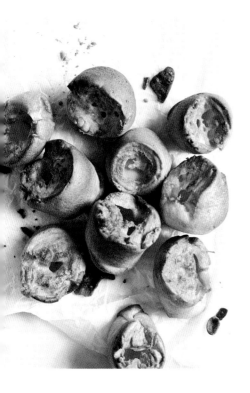

Egg Fried Rice

250g uncooked basmati rice, or
2 x 250g pouches microwave
basmati rice
4 large eggs

2 tbsp tamari sauce
2 tbsp toasted sesame oil
4 spring onions, chopped

Prep: **5 minutes**
Cook: **15 minutes**

DF

It's a no-brainer – egg fried rice is the obvious accompaniment to any of my Chinese-inspired fakeaway dishes, and it's just so easy to make. You can either cook the rice from scratch, or, if feeling lazy (as I often do), you can use pre-cooked microwave pouches instead.
To turn this dish into a full meal, simply stir-fry any meat or veg you choose, then follow the recipe from step two.

Serves 4

1 If making the rice from scratch, add it to a pan containing 500ml boiling water, then cover and cook over a low heat for 10 minutes without lifting the lid. After this time, turn off the heat and leave the lid on for another 5 minutes. After this you can fluff up the rice with a fork, but then cover again and leave to stand for at least 1 hour before using (I often cook it the night before).

2 Place the eggs and tamari in a bowl and beat together lightly.

3 Place the sesame oil in a wok or large frying pan over a medium–high heat. Once hot, add the spring onions and stir-fry for 1–2 minutes.

4 Pour the egg mixture into the wok and stir-fry for another 1–2 minutes, until scrambled. Add the cooked rice straight from the pan or pouches and stir-fry for another 2–3 minutes, until thoroughly hot. Serve alongside your favourite Chinese dishes, such as Sweet & Sour Pork or Chicken & Cashew Nuts (see pages 188 and 189).

Naan Breads

Prep: **1 hour 10 minutes**
Cook: **20 minutes**

EF

120ml warm water
1 tsp caster sugar
7g dried yeast
250g gluten-free white bread
  flour, plus extra for dusting
1 tsp xanthan gum
1 tsp salt

2 tsp nigella seeds
100g natural yoghurt
2 tbsp olive oil

For brushing (optional)
20g butter or ghee
1 tsp crushed garlic

A good curry should always come with a variety of side dishes, and serving your own gluten-free naan bread makes it really special. The dough can be used plain, or flavoured with garlic granules and freshly chopped coriander if you wish. Any leftover naans also make excellent pizza bases when topped with my tomato sauce (see page 180) and grated mozzarella.

Makes 4

1 Place the water in a large jug. Stir in the caster sugar until dissolved, then add the yeast and stir again. Cover with a tea towel and leave in a warm spot for 5–10 minutes to activate the yeast. When ready, it should have a lovely froth on top.

2 Meanwhile, place the flour in a large bowl with the xanthan gum, salt and nigella seeds. Mix well to combine.

3 When the yeast mixture is ready, pour it into the flour along with the yoghurt and olive oil. Mix with a wooden spoon until a sticky dough forms. Cover the bowl with clingfilm and place in a warm spot to prove for 1 hour. The dough will puff up a little but won't double in size.

4 Flour your hands and divide the dough into 4 equal pieces. Roll each one into a ball. Place a sheet of baking paper on a work surface, dust with some extra flour and sit a ball of dough on it. Sprinkle more flour on top, then use your hands to press the dough into a teardrop shape about 1cm thick.

5 Place a dry frying pan over a medium–high heat. When hot, lift the dough off the paper – it should come off easily if you've floured it well – and transfer to the pan. If it sticks to the paper, flip the dough into the pan and then peel off the paper. Cook for 2–3 minutes, until the bread starts to become golden and puff up in places, then flip and cook the other side.

6 Meanwhile, if making the butter and garlic mixture, place the ingredients in a bowl and melt in the microwave.

7 Once the naan bread is cooked, remove from the pan, brush with the garlic butter and wrap in foil, while you repeat the process with the remaining pieces of dough. Serve warm with your favourite curries.

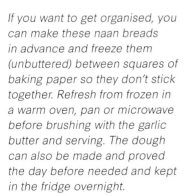

TOP TIP

If you want to get organised, you can make these naan breads in advance and freeze them (unbuttered) between squares of baking paper so they don't stick together. Refresh from frozen in a warm oven, pan or microwave before brushing with the garlic butter and serving. The dough can also be made and proved the day before needed and kept in the fridge overnight.

Garlic & Rosemary Focaccia

250ml water
2 tsp caster sugar
7g dried yeast
250g gluten-free white bread flour, or 220g gluten-free plain flour plus 30g tapioca flour
1 tsp xanthan gum

1 tsp salt
2 tbsp olive oil, plus extra for greasing/drizzling
1 tsp dried rosemary
2 tbsp garlic-infused olive oil
3–4 sprigs of fresh rosemary
Pinch of sea salt flakes

Prep: **1 hour 10 minutes**
Cook: **35 minutes**

EF **DF**

Focaccia is one of the easiest gluten-free breads to make, and, honestly, it tastes divine. Even my gluten-eating friends and family gobble this up as if it's fresh from the bakery. It's incidentally vegan, best eaten warm and perfect for picnics, sharing platters or even dunking in soup. Garlic-infused olive oil gives a subtle but delicious flavour that mingles perfectly with the rosemary.

Makes 1 x 20cm focaccia

1 Measure the water into a heatproof jug and place in the microwave on full power, heating it in 30-second blasts until its temperature hits about 40°C. This should feel like skin temperature if you dip your finger in, but I recommend using a food thermometer to avoid any errors.

2 Stir the sugar into the water until dissolved, then add the yeast and stir again. Cover with a tea towel and leave in a warm spot for 5–10 minutes. When ready, it should have a froth on top.

3 Put the flour, xanthan gum and teaspoon of salt in a bowl and stir to combine. Make a well in the centre and pour in the yeast mixture. Stir with a wooden spoon until it forms a thick batter.

4 Add the measured olive oil, half the garlic-infused olive oil and the dried rosemary. Fold in with the wooden spoon.

5 Use some extra olive oil to generously grease a 20cm round or square baking tin. Scrape in the bread mixture using a spatula, then use oiled fingers to spread it out evenly. Cover loosely with oiled clingfilm and place in a warm, draught-free spot to prove for about 1 hour. In that time, it should have doubled in size.

6 Heat the oven to 220°C/Fan 200°C/Gas Mark 7.

7 Use an oiled thumb or finger to poke dimples in the top of the dough. Arrange the rosemary sprigs on top, then drizzle the remaining tablespoon garlic-infused olive oil over the dough.

8 Bake for 30–35 minutes, until the bread is golden and crisp on top and sounds hollow when tapped. Sprinkle with sea salt flakes and allow to cool for at least 15–30 minutes before removing from the tin and slicing up to serve.

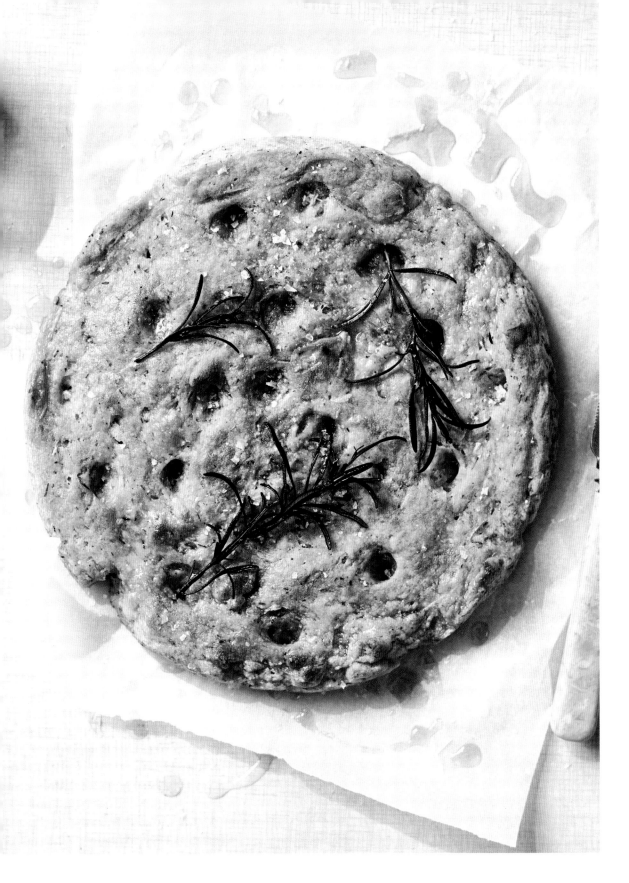

Soda Bread

200ml natural yoghurt
100ml milk
1 tbsp lemon juice
400g gluten-free plain flour, plus extra for dusting

1 tsp salt
1 tbsp caster sugar
½ tsp xanthan gum
2 tsp bicarbonate of soda
1 large egg, lightly whisked

Prep: **15 minutes**
Cook: **30 minutes**

Perfect for serving alongside a soup or stew, this truly simple loaf doesn't require any kneading or proving. The rise comes not from yeast, but from bicarbonate of soda and homemade buttermilk, and the result is a crusty, delicious bread that is best eaten warm and slathered in butter. Everyone will be super-impressed you made it, so don't tell them it's a doddle.

Serves 6-8

1   Preheat the oven to 190ºC/Fan 170ºC/Gas Mark 5. Line a baking sheet with baking paper and set aside.

2   Place the yoghurt, milk and lemon juice in a bowl and mix well. The lemon juice should cause the mixture to curdle a little, forming buttermilk.

3   Place the flour in a large bowl with the salt, sugar, xanthan gum and bicarbonate of soda. Mix well, then pour in your buttermilk and the egg, and mix with a wooden spoon to form a soft, sticky dough.

4   Dust your work surface with a little extra flour and turn the dough onto it. Dust your hands with flour too, then lightly shape the dough into a ball. The extra flour will make it more workable, but take care not to add too much, and don't overwork it – you don't want the dough to be super-stiff.

5   Flatten the dough into a circle about 20cm wide. It should hold its shape quite well, but might spread a little, so don't worry if it does. Place on the prepared baking sheet and use a sharp knife to score an X on the top.

6   Sprinkle with a little extra flour, then bake in the centre of the oven for about 30 minutes. The loaf should be lovely and golden, and sound hollow when tapped on the top and bottom. Transfer to a wire rack to cool for at least 30 minutes before slicing and serving.

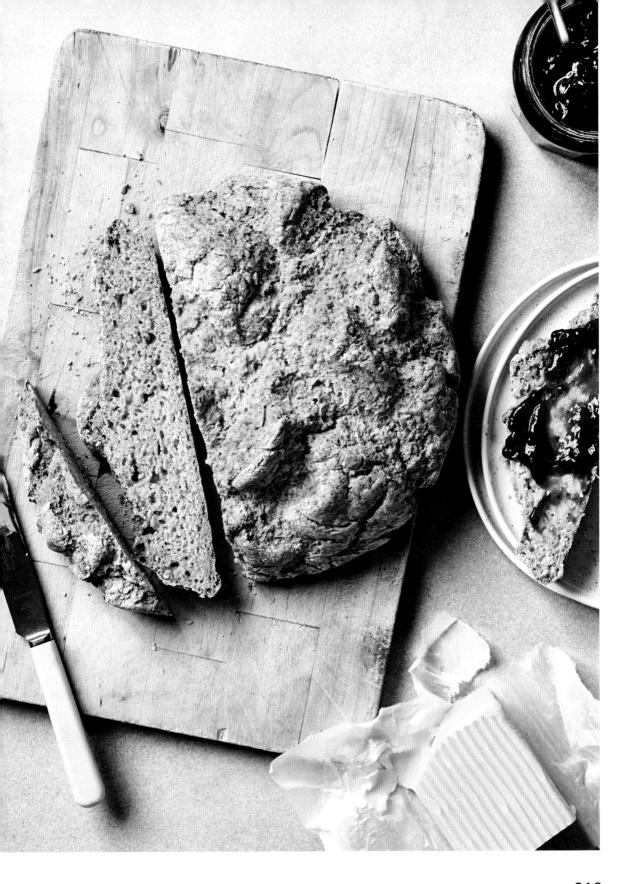

Cheesy Dough Balls

300g gluten-free plain flour
3 tsp baking powder
¼ tsp xanthan gum
300g natural yoghurt or
    dairy-free alternative

75g mature Cheddar or
    dairy-free alternative, grated
20g salted butter, melted
½ tsp garlic paste
Handful of fresh parsley,
    chopped

Prep: **10 minutes**
Cook: **20 minutes**

I couldn't create a recipe book without including the cheesy dough balls that accompany most of my own dinners. This simple side dish was born out of sheer boredom during the lockdown of 2020, and has been one of the most popular recipes on my blog ever since. I'm not sure if it's the doughy deliciousness or the fact you could pretty much make them with your eyes shut, but I apologise in advance if you simply cannot stop eating them.

Makes 12

1   Preheat the oven to 200°C/Fan 180°C/Gas Mark 6. Line a baking tray with baking paper.

2   Combine the flour, baking powder and xanthan gum in a large bowl, then add the yoghurt and cheese. Stir with a spoon or spatula until the mixture thickens. At that point, use your hands to bring it all together into a smooth and slightly sticky dough.

3   Break the dough into 12 equal pieces (about 50g each). Roll them into balls and space them out on the prepared tray.

4   Bake for 15–20 minutes, until golden on top.

5   Mix the melted butter, garlic paste and parsley together in a small bowl and either brush this over the hot dough balls as soon as they come out of the oven, or serve it as a dip for them alongside your favourite pizza or pasta dish.

TOP TIP

If you want to make this recipe dairy-free or vegan, I recommend using coconut yoghurt and a good-quality dairy-free cheese. You honestly wouldn't know the difference.

Garlic Pizza Bread

Gluten-free plain flour, for dusting
½ quantity pizza dough (see page 180)
40g butter or dairy-free alternative
3 tsp chopped garlic
½ tsp dried rosemary
½ tsp salt

Prep: **1¼ hours**
Cook: **30 minutes**

If ever I'm making a pasta dish, garlic bread is an obligatory accompaniment, and sometimes, just for a change, I make it with pizza dough. Easy to make and perfect for sharing, just slice it up, stack it high and offer alongside any pasta or risotto dish. In fact, serve it with whatever you fancy. I will eat garlic pizza bread with literally anything, for any meal, and can often be found snaffling leftovers from the fridge for a snack.

Makes 1 x 30cm pizza base

1 When the dough has proved, preheat the oven to 240ºC/Fan 220ºC/Gas Mark 9. Also set out a pizza mesh or a non-stick baking sheet.

2 Place a 35cm length of baking paper on your work surface and dust it with a little flour. If you want to make a precise pizza shape, you can draw around a dinner plate on the paper to use as a guide, or just freestyle it. Dust your hands so that the dough doesn't stick to them, then place it on the floured paper and gently push it into a circular shape about 1–2cm thick and 30cm across.

3 Place a pizza mesh (if you have one) over the dough, then carefully lift the baking paper and flip it over so that the dough is sitting on the mesh. Alternatively, invert the pizza base onto a non-stick baking sheet. Carefully peel off the baking paper.

4 Place the butter in a bowl and melt in the microwave. Mix in the garlic, rosemary and salt.

5 Spoon the butter mixture onto the pizza base, then use a pastry brush to spread it evenly, leaving a clear 1cm border around the perimeter.

6 Bake for 15–20 minutes, until golden around the edges, then serve with your favourite dishes.

Sweet Potato Samosas

Prep: **45 minutes**
Cook: **15 minutes**

I'd actually never tried a samosa before going gluten free, so finally creating my own was a dream come true. These lovely little mouthfuls are one of those foods you don't realise you're missing out on until you can't eat one – so now I like to whip up a batch and keep them in the freezer so I can join in when everyone else gets a takeaway curry. They're also a great idea for lunches – just reheat in the oven and you're good to go.

150ml warm water
1 tbsp whole psyllium husks
200g gluten-free plain flour
30g tapioca flour
1 tsp xanthan gum
½ tsp salt
370ml vegetable oil
1 egg, beaten

For the filling
1 tbsp vegetable oil
250g sweet potato, chopped into 1cm cubes
1 red onion, finely chopped
75g frozen peas
1 tsp chopped garlic
1 tsp ginger paste
1 tsp mild curry powder
100ml gluten-free vegetable stock

Makes 8

1   Start by making the filling. Heat the oil in a large frying pan and add the sweet potato, red onion and frozen peas. Fry for 5 minutes over a medium heat, then add the garlic, ginger paste and curry powder. Stir well and fry for another 30 seconds. Pour in the stock, mix well and cover the pan with a lid. Turn the heat to low and cook for 20 minutes, stirring once or twice, until the potato has softened. Remove the lid, take off the heat and leave to cool while you make the pastry as per steps 1–2 on page 218.

2   Divide the pastry into 8 equal pieces and roll each of them into a ball. Place all but one of them on a board and wrap in clingfilm to stop them from drying out.

3   Place a 35cm length of clingfilm on your work surface and sit the unwrapped ball of pastry on it. Press with your hand to flatten it, cover with another sheet of clingfilm, then use a rolling pin to roll the dough into a circle about 15cm in diameter. Remove the top sheet of clingfilm.

4   Divide the filling into 8 equal portions of about 2 tablespoons. Place one portion in the centre of the circle, then brush around the edges of the pastry with the beaten egg.

5   Now fold the dough into a triangle shape: using the clingfilm to help you, fold the right-hand side of the dough over the filling towards the middle. Then fold the left-hand side over to the middle, forming a point at the top. Finally, fold up the bottom of the dough to close the triangle, then press together any open corners. Repeat the rolling, filling and folding with the remaining pieces of dough.

6   Pour a 1–2 cm depth of the remaining oil into a saucepan and heat to 200ºC, or until a small cube of bread browns in 10 seconds. Fry the samosas in small batches for 2–3 minutes on each side, until golden. Transfer to a plate lined with kitchen paper to drain before serving with your favourite curry dishes.

Beautiful Bhajis

1 tbsp vegetable oil, plus extra
  for deep-frying
3 large onions, finely sliced
1 tsp chilli powder
½ tsp cumin seeds
¼ tsp ground turmeric

For the batter
100g gram (chickpea) flour
Pinch of salt
½ tsp ground cumin
100ml cold water

Prep: **10 minutes**
Cook: **20 minutes**

Even though onion bhajis are traditionally made with gram (chickpea) flour, which is naturally gluten free, those sold in supermarkets and takeaways are not. Making your own is the best way to combat this – plus it's actually a lot easier than you think.

Makes 8

1. Place the tablespoon of oil in a large frying pan over a low heat. Once hot, add the onions and fry, stirring frequently, for 6–8 minutes, until they have softened.

2. Add the chilli powder, cumin seeds and turmeric, mix well and fry for another minute. Remove the pan from the heat.

3. Place all the batter ingredients in a large bowl and beat together until smooth. Add the onion mixture and stir well.

4. Pour a 1cm depth of extra oil into a pan and place over a high heat until a food thermometer registers 200ºC or a tiny bit of batter dropped into it floats to the surface and bubbles form around it.

5. Gently lower 2-tablespoon heaps of the onion mixture into the oil. Press down slightly, and fry for 2 minutes on each side, until golden brown. Transfer to a plate lined with kitchen paper and keep warm. Fry the remaining onion mixture in the same way. Serve the bhajis with your favourite curries.

TOP TIP

If you want a lower-fat version of these samosas, you can bake them in a hot oven (200ºC/ Fan 180ºC/Gas Mark 6) for 20 minutes rather than frying them, but they won't become as crisp and crunchy.

Vegetable Spring Rolls

Prep: **45 minutes**
Cook: **15 minutes**

DF

When I first decided to develop a spring roll recipe, I wasn't sure I'd even know if I got them right, given it had been at least two decades since I had a 'normal' one. But when I had a bite of these, it took me right back. These are the perfect side dish for a Chinese fakeaway. Try adding cooked chicken or prawns if you like to mix them up a bit. Any leftovers can be frozen, and I recommend reheating them in the oven once defrosted so they stay crisp.

150ml warm water
1 tbsp whole psyllium husks
200g gluten-free plain flour, plus extra for dusting
30g tapioca flour
1 tsp xanthan gum
½ tsp salt
370ml vegetable oil
1 egg, beaten

For the filling
50g gluten-free vermicelli rice noodles
1 tbsp toasted sesame oil
300g stir-fry vegetable mixture, such as peppers, carrots, cabbage, beansprouts
1½ tbsp tamari sauce

Makes 12

1 Place the warm water in a bowl, add the psyllium husks and mix well until a gel-like consistency begins to form. Leave for 1 minute.

2 Place both flours in a bowl with the xanthan gum and salt. Pour in the psyllium gel, add 4 teaspoons of the oil and mix with a wooden spoon until the mixture becomes claggy. Now use your hands to 'squish' it into a slightly sticky dough, and knead until it forms a smooth ball. Wrap tightly in clingfilm and leave to rest at room temperature while you move on to the next step.

3 To make the filling, bring a pan of water to the boil, then add the rice noodles. Turn off the heat, cover with a lid and leave for 4–5 minutes, before draining.

4 Meanwhile, heat the sesame oil in a wok or large frying pan over a medium–high heat. Once hot, add the vegetables and tamari and stir-fry for 2–3 minutes.

5 Add the drained noodles and continue to stir-fry for another minute.

6 Spread the noodle mixture over a large plate and leave to cool for 10 minutes.

7 To construct the spring rolls, divide the wrapper dough into 12 equal pieces, about 30–35g each. Place all but one of them on a board, wrap in clingfilm and set aside.

8 Place a 35cm length of baking paper on your work surface and lightly dust with extra flour. Sit the unwrapped ball of dough on the paper and use your hand to flatten it down. Dust lightly with extra flour, then place another sheet of

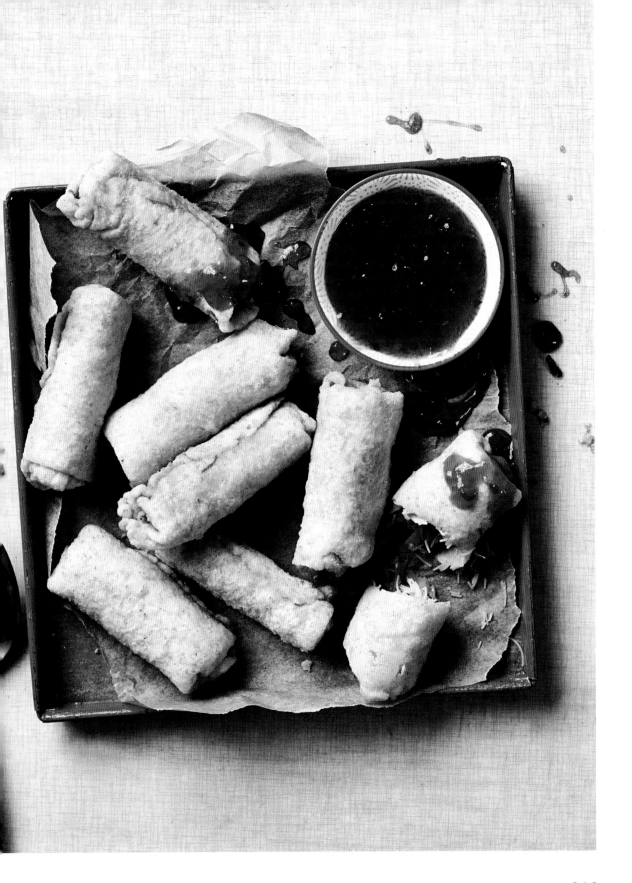

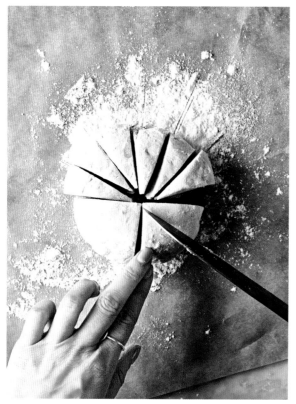

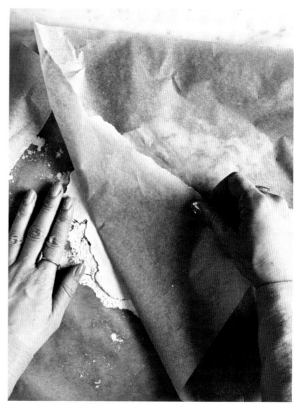

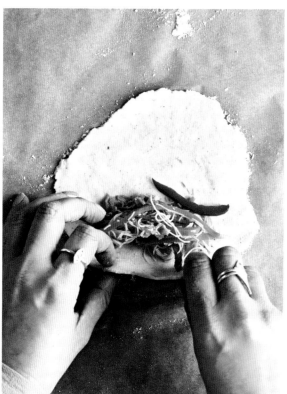

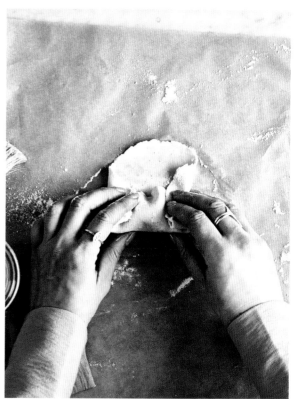

BITS ON THE SIDE

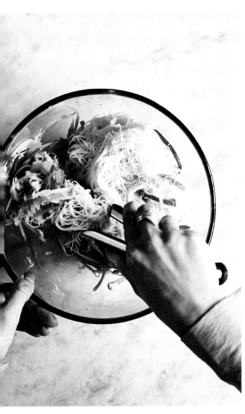

baking paper on top and use a rolling pin to roll the dough into a circle about 15cm in diameter, turning it regularly to ensure it's even. Remove the top sheet of baking paper.

9 Divide the filling into roughly 12 equal portions, and place one portion in a line in the middle of the wrapper, leaving a 2.5cm space all around it.

10 Place the wrapper so the filling is running parallel to the edge of the work surface. Fold the side closest to you over the filling, then curve your fingers around it and pull back slightly to tuck the wrap underneath. Fold in the sides, then brush the open edge with beaten egg before folding over and rolling into a tight cylinder. Repeat steps 8–10 to make 12 spring rolls in total. Transfer them to a plate and cover with clingfilm to stop them from drying out.

11 Heat a 1cm depth of the vegetable oil in a large frying pan until it reaches 190ºC, or a small cube of bread browns in 10 seconds. Add the spring rolls a few at a time to ensure there is about 2.5cm between them and fry for 2 minutes. Turn them over and fry for another 2 minutes. Transfer to a plate lined with kitchen paper and keep warm. Cook the remaining spring rolls in the same way, then serve hot alongside your favourite fakeaway dishes.

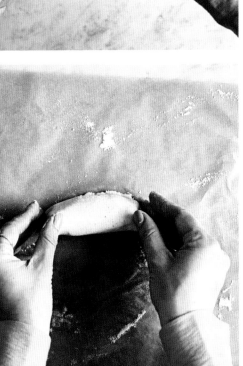

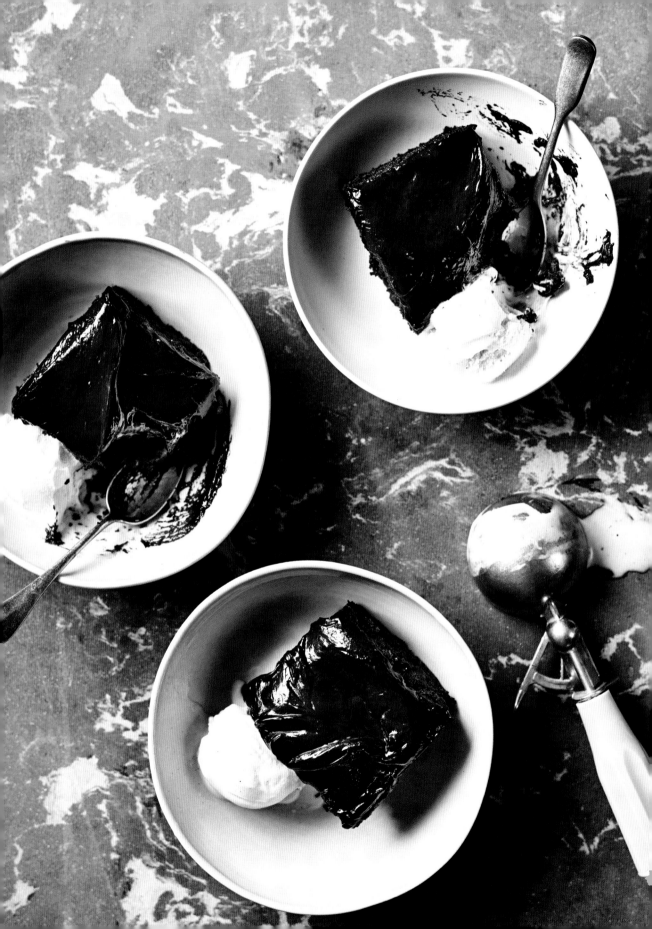

DESSERTS

If there's one thing you won't find in this dessert section, it's a fruit salad. For too long we gluten-free folk have suffered boring and sparse dessert menus – but no more! Sometimes you just need a sweet treat to finish off your meal, whether that's a sharing dessert or a cheeky little something for one. There are plenty of options in this chapter to suit every dessert fan.

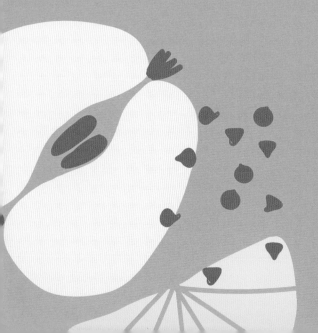

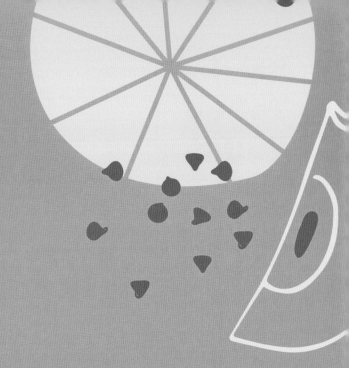

Sticky Toffee Pudding

Prep: **20 minutes**
Cook: **40 minutes**

200g Medjool dates, stones
  removed
250ml boiling water
½ tsp vanilla extract
50g unsalted butter, plus extra
  for greasing
100g dark brown sugar
50g caster sugar
2 large eggs

200g gluten-free self-raising
  flour
1½ tsp bicarbonate of soda

For the sauce
130g unsalted butter
1 tsp vanilla extract
150g dark brown sugar
200ml double cream

I've never been a huge dessert person, but there's nothing like watching someone devour a sticky toffee pudding in a restaurant to fill you with food envy. Not any more! This recipe for sticky toffee pudding is all my gluten-free prayers come true, not least because I could simply bathe in a vat of the toffee sauce and be happy forever.

Serves 8

1   Finely chop the dates. Place in a saucepan with the boiling water and vanilla extract and bring to the boil. Simmer for 2–3 minutes, then set aside to cool for about 10 minutes before you make the cake batter.

2   Preheat the oven to 180°C/Fan 160°C/Gas Mark 4. Grease a 30 x 20cm baking dish with the extra butter.

3   To make the batter, place the butter and sugars in a bowl and beat with an electric whisk for 1–2 minutes. Add the eggs and beat again, until combined. Sift in the flour and bicarbonate of soda and beat for another minute.

4   Using a spatula, fold in the dates until fully combined.

5   Pour the batter into the prepared dish and bake in the centre of the oven for 30–35 minutes, until the cake starts to come away from the sides. Set aside to cool slightly.

6   Meanwhile, to make the sauce, place the butter, vanilla extract and sugar in a large pan over a low heat, stirring regularly until the butter has melted and the sugar has dissolved. Add the cream, bring to the boil and simmer for 1–2 minutes.

7   Pour the sauce over the warm cake and serve straight away. For extra indulgence, the pudding can also be served with custard, cream or ice-cream.

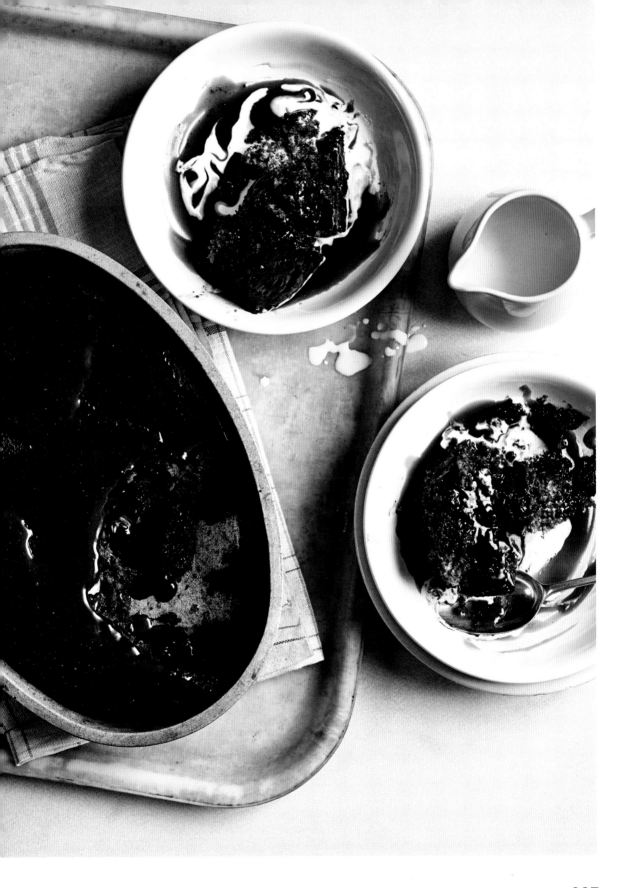

Citrus Meringue Pie

Prep: **15 minutes**
Cook: **30 minutes**

Lemon meringue pie might well have been my favourite dessert of all time...until I tried adding orange and grapefruit to the mix. With buttery pastry, a tangy citrus curd filling and pillowy meringue, this dessert is a true delight that everyone will enjoy. Don't you just want to face-plant that meringue?

Gluten-free plain flour,
  for dusting
½ quantity chilled Shortcrust
  Pastry (see page 39)

For the citrus curd
4 medium eggs, plus 1 large egg
Juice of 1 grapefruit
Juice of 1 orange
Zest and juice of 2 lemons

65g cornflour
250g caster sugar
85g unsalted butter

For the meringue
4 egg whites, reserved from
  above
200g caster sugar
2 tsp cornflour

Serves 12

1   Preheat the oven to 180ºC/Fan 160ºC/Gas Mark 4.

2   Flour a clean work surface and roll the pastry into a circle about 4mm thick. Use it to line a deep, 23cm fluted pie tin, gently pressing it into the sides. Fold the overhanging pastry back over the rim to make the edge slightly thicker (which minimises shrinking), then run your rolling pin over the tin to remove any excess pastry. Prick all over the bottom of the pastry case with a fork and blind bake as described on page 39.

3   Meanwhile, make the curd filling. Separate the 4 medium eggs into 2 bowls. Add the whole large egg to the yolks and beat together.

4   Place all the citrus juices in a jug and put the cornflour in a bowl. Add the juice to the cornflour a little at a time, stirring until a smooth paste forms. (You will not need all the juice for this.)

5   Place the caster sugar and butter in a saucepan along with the cornflour paste, lemon zest and the remaining juice. Bring to a simmer over a low heat , stirring constantly with a whisk, for 1–2 minutes, then take off the heat. Add the egg yolk mixture and beat vigorously with a wooden spoon for another minute. Set to one side.

6   To make the meringue, beat the reserved egg whites in a large bowl with an electric whisk until they form soft peaks. Continue to whisk while adding the caster sugar a tablespoon at a time, beating between each addition. Sprinkle in the cornflour and beat for another 30 seconds, until glossy peaks form.

7   Pour the citrus curd into the baked pastry case and spread smoothly. Spoon dollops of the meringue around the perimeter of the curd – if you put it in the middle first, it might sink – then

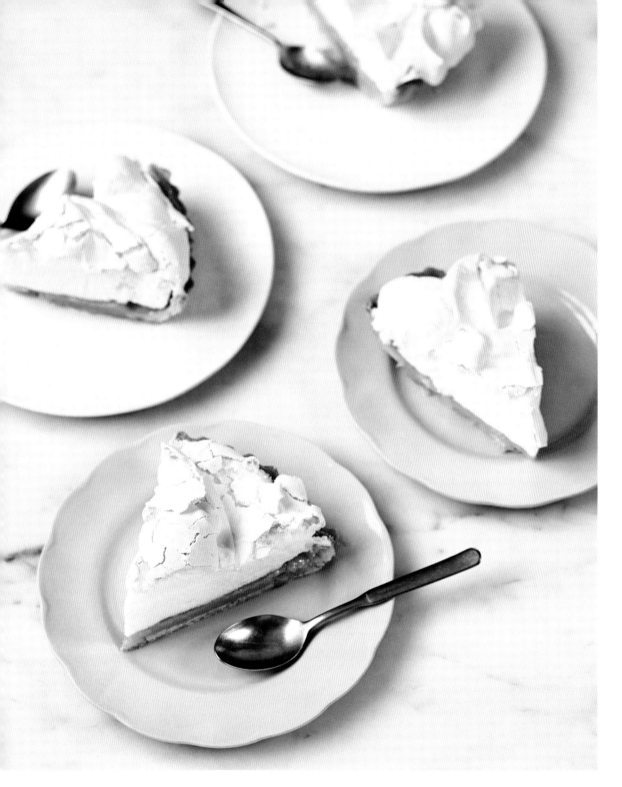

spread the meringue into the fluted edges. Pile the rest of the meringue into the middle and swirl it with a fork.

8   Bake the pie for 15–20 minutes, until the meringue is golden. Set aside to cool completely before serving.

Chocolate Fudge Cake

Prep: **10 minutes**
Cook: **35 minutes**

I always like to have an 'emergency dessert' in the freezer, and this chocolate fudge traybake is perfect. You can portion it up and freeze it, ready for those moments when it's a case of life or death on the chocolate front. It can be enjoyed as a straightforward cake, but zap it in the microwave so that the frosting turns into a gorgeous fudge sauce, and you have a dessert classic on your plate.

Butter, for greasing
100g dark chocolate
175g gluten-free self-raising flour
30g cocoa powder
150ml vegetable oil
100ml buttermilk
175g caster sugar
3 large eggs

¼ tsp xanthan gum

For the chocolate ganache
150g dark chocolate, finely chopped
150g milk chocolate, finely chopped
150ml double cream

Makes 16 Squares

1 Preheat the oven to 180°C/Fan 160°C/Gas Mark 4. Grease a 24cm square cake tin and line it with baking paper.

2 To make the cake, break the dark chocolate into pieces and melt on full power in the microwave in 10-second bursts. Set aside to cool a little.

3 Meanwhile, place the flour and all the remaining cake ingredients in a large bowl and beat together with an electric whisk until fully combined. Pour in the cooled, melted chocolate and fold into the mixture.

4 Pour the batter into the prepared tin, smooth the top and bake for 25–30 minutes, until the top bounces back when gently pressed with a finger, or a skewer inserted in the middle comes out clean.

5 Transfer to a cooling rack for 10–15 minutes, then remove the cake from the tin. Peel off the baking paper and leave to cool completely.

6 When you're ready to top the cake, place all the chopped chocolate in a large bowl.

7 Pour the double cream into a small saucepan over a very low heat until it just starts to simmer. Don't let it get to a full boil. Pour the hot cream over the chocolate and mix until smooth. Allow to cool for about 10 minutes.

8 Spread the cooled ganache evenly over the top of the cake. Leave to set.

9 Serve as a treat whenever you feel like it, or heat as suggested above when you want a warm fudgy dessert.

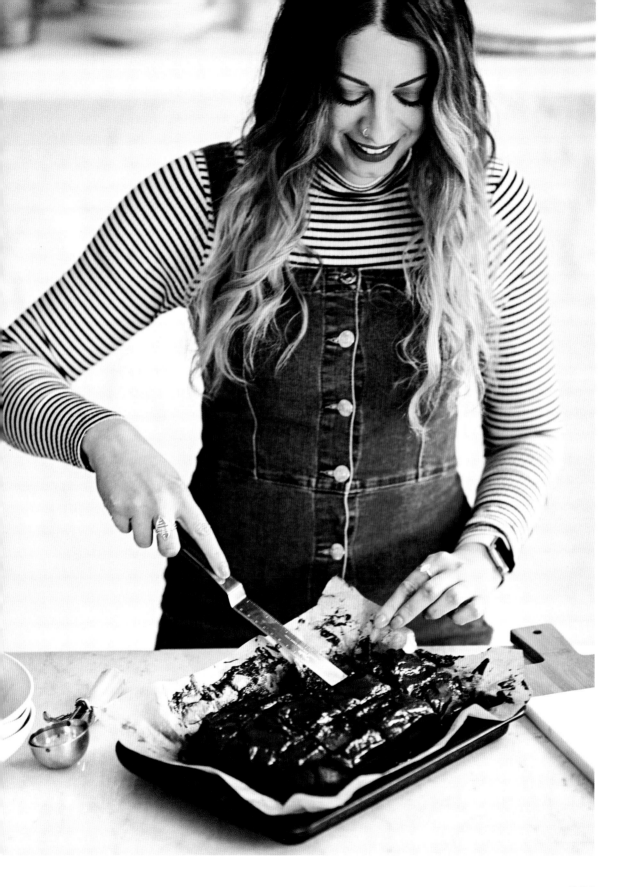

Toffee Apple Pie

800g Bramley apples
50g dark brown sugar
30g unsalted butter
Juice of ½ lemon
2 tbsp cornflour
1 tsp ground cinnamon

150g dulce de leche
Gluten-free flour, for dusting
1 quantity chilled Shortcrust
 Pastry (see page 39)
1 egg, beaten
2 tbsp granulated sugar

Prep: **30 minutes**
Cook: **50 minutes**

If you thought you loved apple pie, wait to fall in love all over again with my gluten-free toffee apple pie. It has all the traditional ingredients – gluten free, of course – so you can still enjoy the buttery pastry and tart apple chunks, but the addition of caramel takes it to a whole new level. The only question is...ice-cream or custard on top?

Serves 6

1 Peel, core and quarter the apples, then cut each quarter into 5mm slices. Add them to a large pan along with the dark brown sugar, butter, lemon juice, cornflour and cinnamon. Place over a low heat and cook, stirring frequently, for 10–12 minutes, until the apples have softened and any liquid in the pan has thickened.

2 Take the pan off the heat, stir in the dulce de leche and set to one side.

3 Preheat the oven to 180°C/Fan 160°C/Gas Mark 5.

4 Lightly dust a work surface with flour, then roll the chilled pastry into a circle about 4mm thick. Use it to line a 23cm pie dish, then trim off the excess. Prick the bottom of the pastry case several times with a fork, then brush the edges with beaten egg.

5 Pour the apple filling into the pie dish and spread evenly.

6 Scrunch the pastry offcuts together and reroll to about 4mm thick. Cut into strips around 2.5cm wide, then lay them across the top of the pie in a lattice pattern. Press the edges together with your fingers and trim off any excess. Crimp the edges using a fork.

7 Brush the pastry with beaten egg and sprinkle with the granulated sugar. Bake for 45–50 minutes, until golden. Set aside for 30 minutes before serving with custard or ice-cream.

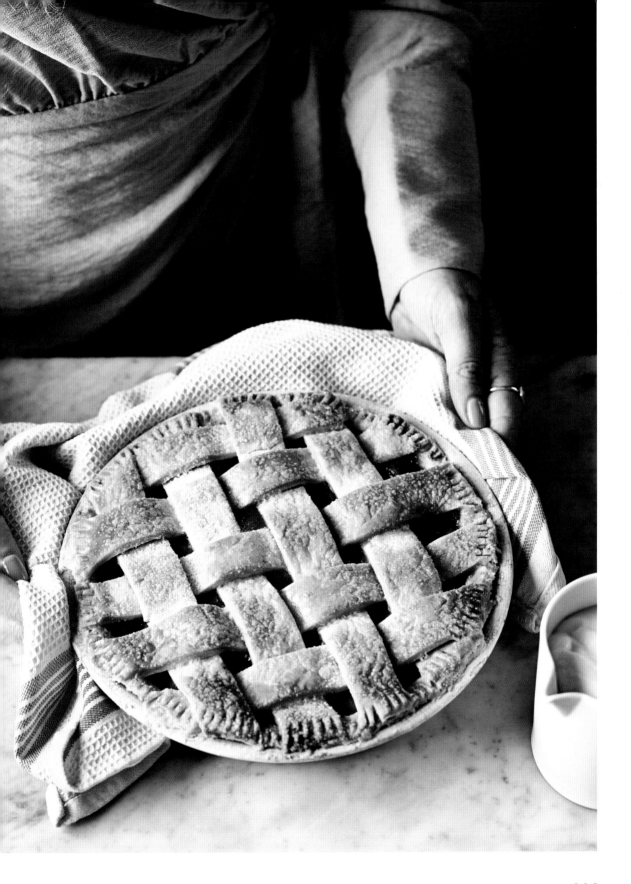

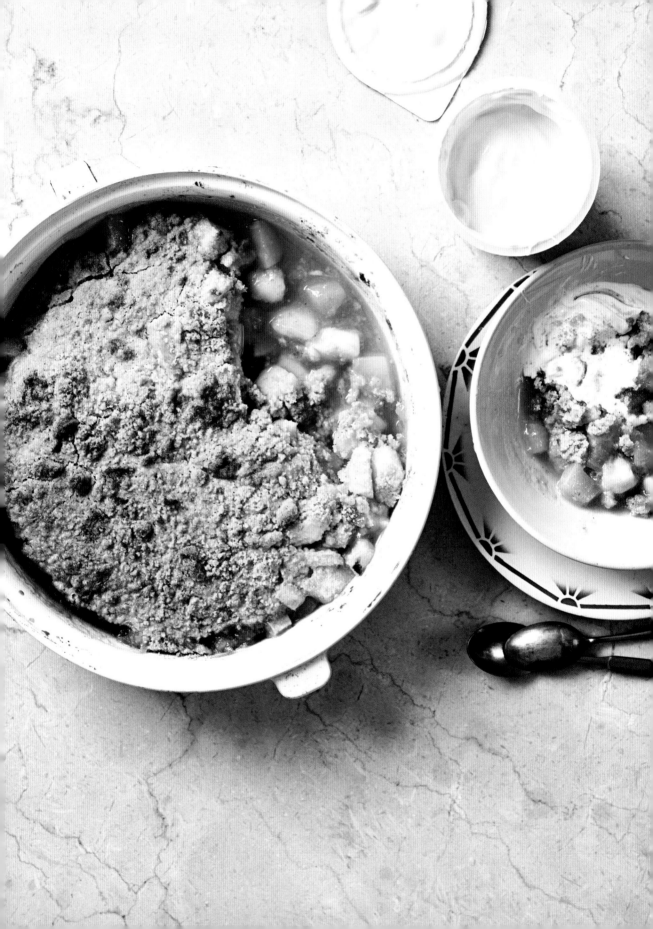

Pear & Ginger Crumble

150g gluten-free plain flour
1½ tsp baking powder
1 tsp ground ginger
75g caster sugar
75g unsalted butter,
  cut into 1cm cubes

For the filling
6 Conference pears
125g stem ginger in syrup, diced
1 tbsp light brown sugar

Prep: **10 minutes**
Cook: **50 minutes**

EF

You might have heard that certain gluten-free foods have a reputation for being crumbly, but that quality comes into its own here to make an exceptional crumble topping. This five-ingredient topping can be generously draped over any fruit filling, but I absolutely adore it with sticky pears and stem ginger.

Serves 6

1 Preheat the oven to 180°C/Fan 160°C/Gas Mark 4.

2 To make the filling, peel, quarter and core the pears, then cut them into 1–2cm chunks. You want enough to thickly cover the base of a 20cm pie dish.

3 Place the pear chunks in the dish, then add the stem ginger and brown sugar. Mix well until both are evenly distributed, then set to one side.

4 To make the crumble, place the flour, baking powder, ground ginger, caster sugar and butter in a large bowl. Use your fingers to rub the mix together until it forms a breadcrumb consistency. Pour the crumble over the fruit, making sure there are no gaps.

5 Bake for 45–50 minutes, until the crumble is golden brown and the fruit is bubbling underneath. You want the fruit to be soft but with a little bite. Serve hot with custard or ice-cream.

Baked New York Cheesecake

200g gluten-free digestive biscuits
25g caster sugar
75g unsalted butter, melted

For the topping
650g full-fat cream cheese
150g soured cream
175g caster sugar
3 large eggs
1 tsp vanilla extract
45g gluten-free plain flour

Prep: **20 minutes**
Cook: **55 minutes (+ 8 hours cooling)**

With a buttery base and the creamiest topping, this cheesecake will be popular with literally everyone. In fact, it's so good that I defy anyone to identify it as gluten free. Serve it up with fresh berries on top, or a drizzle of chocolate or caramel sauce for extra pizzazz.

Serves 12

1 Preheat the oven to 180°C/Fan 160°C/Gas Mark 5. Unclip the base of a 20cm springform tin, cover tightly with a sheet of baking paper, then clip it back into the tin. Trim off any excess paper around the edges, then wrap the outside of the whole tin in a sheet of foil – this will catch any leaks that might happen during baking. Set to one side.

2 Place the digestives and sugar in a food processor and blitz into crumbs. Pour in the melted butter and blitz again to combine.

3 Tip the biscuit mixture into the prepared tin and press it down in a smooth layer on the bottom (and a little up the sides if you like). Bake for 10 minutes, then set aside.

4 Increase the oven temperature to 220°C/Fan 200°C/Gas Mark 7. Place a roasting tray in the bottom of the oven and add a 2.5–5cm depth of boiling water: the steam from it will help to prevent the cheesecake from cracking.

5 To make the filling, place the cream cheese, soured cream and sugar in a large bowl and beat with an electric whisk for 1–2 minutes, until smooth.

6 Crack the eggs into a separate bowl and beat lightly to combine. Add the vanilla extract to the cream cheese, then add a third of the egg mixture. Beat for 30 seconds, then add another third of the eggs. Beat again and repeat with the remainder of the eggs.

7 Sprinkle the flour into the filling mixture and beat for 1 minute, until smooth.

8 Pour the filling over the biscuit base, then bake for 10 minutes.

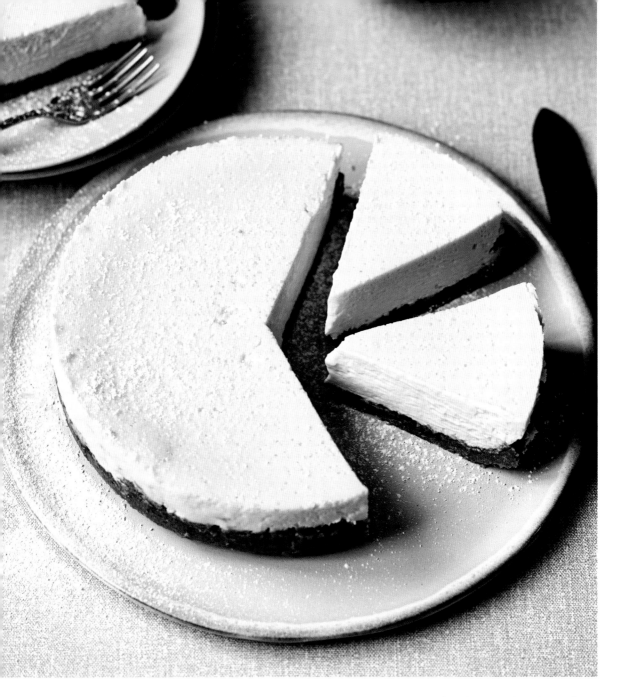

After this time, and without opening the oven door, lower the temperature to 110ºC/Fan 90ºC/Gas Mark ¼. Bake for a further 45 minutes, by which time the cheesecake should wobble a little but not look liquid. If the centre still looks very 'sloshy', give it another 5–10 minutes.

9 When ready, turn the oven off and, keeping the door closed, leave the cheesecake inside for 2 hours to cool. After that, transfer to the fridge and leave overnight, or for at least 6 hours, before serving.

Sharing Skillet Cookie

90g butter, melted, plus extra for greasing
40g granulated sugar
120g light brown sugar
1 egg
1 tsp vanilla extract

220g gluten-free plain flour
½ tsp bicarbonate of soda
¼ tsp xanthan gum
¼ tsp salt
150g mixture of milk and white chocolate chips

Prep: **5 minutes**

Cook: **30 minutes**
(+ 20 minutes resting)

Does anything say 'cosy night in' more than wrapping up in a blanket, chucking on a good movie and diving into a warm chocolatey cookie with ice-cream? This giant sharing cookie, made in what Americans call a skillet and we call a frying pan, has a decadent, gooey centre and melty chocolate chunks, and it's honestly the epitome of comfort food. Mix it up with toffee chunks, chopped nuts or dark chocolate if you like.

Serves 4

1 Preheat the oven to 200ºC/Fan 180ºC/Gas Mark 6. Lightly grease a 20cm ovenproof frying pan with extra butter and set to one side.

2 Place the melted butter and sugars in a bowl and beat with an electric whisk for 1 minute. Add the egg and vanilla extract and beat for another 30 seconds.

3 Combine the flour, bicarb, xanthan gum and salt in a separate bowl, then add to the egg mixture along with the chocolate chips. Stir with a wooden spoon until a thick dough forms and there's no loose flour.

4 Turn the dough into the prepared pan. Wet your hands, so the dough doesn't stick to them, and press it down in an even layer.

5 Bake for 20 minutes, until golden on top. This will result in a gorgeous, gooey centre, but, if you prefer a firmer cookie, bake for another 5–10 minutes. Allow to sit for 15–20 minutes before tucking into the warm cookie with spoons straight from the pan. Add a dollop of ice-cream if you like.

TOP TIP

No ovenproof frying pan? Simply use a 20cm baking tin instead. You can always cut the cookie into bars or wedges before serving if you find that easier.

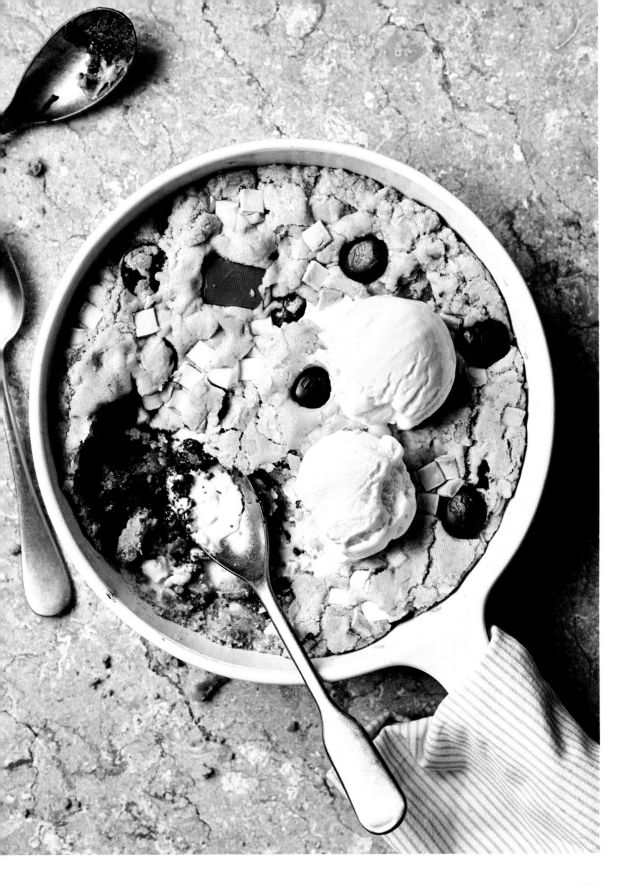

Chocolate Stuffed Pancakes

with Caramelised Bananas

8 tsp chocolate spread
1 large egg
225g milk
100ml buttermilk
200g gluten-free plain flour
2½ tsp baking powder
¼ tsp xanthan gum
1 tbsp caster sugar
Butter, for frying

For the caramelised bananas
2 bananas
80g caster sugar
40g unsalted butter

Prep: **15 minutes**
(+ 1 hour freezing)

Cook: **25 minutes**

Fluffy American pancakes are always a thing of joy, but it doesn't get much more decadent than stuffing them with melting chocolate spread. That is, of course, until you also top them with sticky, caramelised bananas. Forget just saving this recipe for a pudding – it's about to become your new breakfast/brunch/weekend treat/need-dessert-for-dinner favourite.

Makes 8

1   Place a sheet of baking paper on a baking tray or chopping board and put a teaspoonful of chocolate spread on it. Use the back of the spoon to spread it into a disc about 5cm wide and 5mm thick. Repeat until you have 8 discs, then pop them in the freezer for at least 1 hour.

2   When the chocolate discs are frozen, start making the pancakes. Place the egg, milk and buttermilk in a jug and mix together with a whisk.

3   Place the flour in a bowl with the baking powder, xanthan gum and caster sugar. Stir to combine, then add to the jug, whisking until smooth.

4   Melt a knob of butter in a non-stick frying pan over a medium heat. Meanwhile, take 2 chocolate discs out of the freezer; I do this in batches of 2 as they soften very quickly.

5   Swirl the butter around the pan, then pour in 2 half-ladles of batter, leaving plenty of space between them. Note: if you pour the batter from a height of 5–7.5cm above the pan, it spreads into a more even shape. Place a chocolate disc on each pancake, then pour another 1–2 tablespoons of batter on top to cover the chocolate completely. Cook for about 2 minutes, until little bubbles start to form on top of the pancakes, then flip them over and cook for another 2 minutes. You want them to be golden brown so, if they start to smoke or cook too quickly, turn the heat down.

6   Transfer to an ovenproof dish, cover with foil and place in a low oven to keep warm. Repeat steps 4, 5 and 6 to make

TOP TIP

Did you know you can freeze these pancakes? Simply cool them, stack between sheets of baking paper so they don't stick together, and place in a plastic container. Defrost and reheat in the microwave or frying pan for an easy dessert on demand.

240

DESSERTS

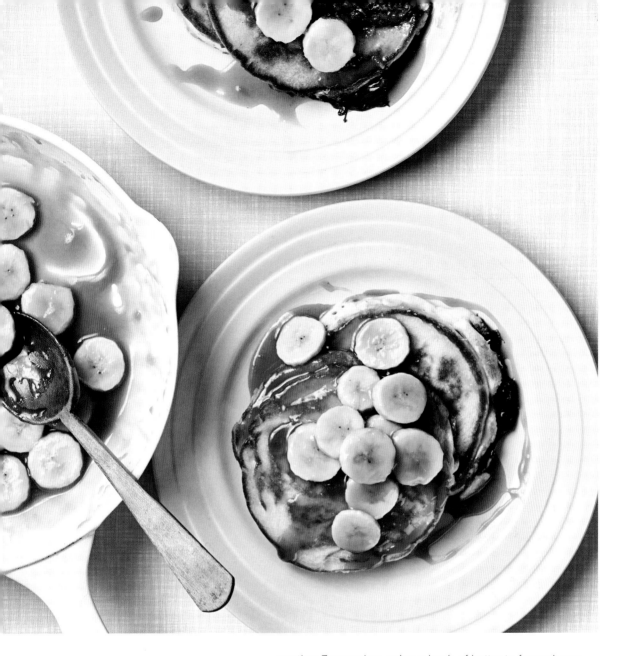

another 7 pancakes, using a knob of butter to fry each one.

7 While the final pancakes are cooking, peel the bananas and slice them into discs about 1cm thick.

8 Place a clean frying pan over a low heat and add the caster sugar, stirring occasionally with a wooden spoon for 1–2 minutes, until it has melted and started to brown.

9 Take off the heat, add the butter and stir well. Place the banana discs in the caramel, then return the pan to a low heat. Cook for 1–2 minutes on each side, then serve on top of the pancakes.

No-Bake Chocolate Orange Tart

300g gluten-free digestive
  biscuits
30g cocoa powder
100g unsalted butter, melted

For the filling
150g dark chocolate, plus extra
  for grating

150g milk chocolate
50g unsalted butter, cut into
  small cubes
2 tsp orange extract
300ml double cream
Zest of 1 orange

Prep: **30 minutes**
(+ 4 hours chilling)

EF

I love a no-bake dessert – even more so when it looks like you've been slaving away in the kitchen for hours. In reality, you can have this tart thrown together in less than half an hour, and then stashed in the fridge, ready for your guests. Make it the night before you need it for extra ease.

Serves 12

1 Place the digestives and cocoa powder in a food processor and blitz into crumbs. Add the melted butter and blitz again so it forms a consistency like wet sand.

2 Tip the biscuit mixture into a deep, 23cm loose-bottomed tart tin. Spread it out with your hands, taking it up the sides too, then press it down firmly; the base of a tumbler is good for this. Place in the freezer while you make the filling.

3 Place the chopped chocolate in a bowl with the butter and the orange extract.

4 Heat the cream in a pan until just before boiling point. Pour it over the chocolate and mix until smooth.

5 Remove the base from the freezer and pour in the filling. Smooth it out with a spatula, then chill overnight, or for at least 4 hours.

6 Decorate with the orange zest and a sprinkling of finely grated chocolate before serving.

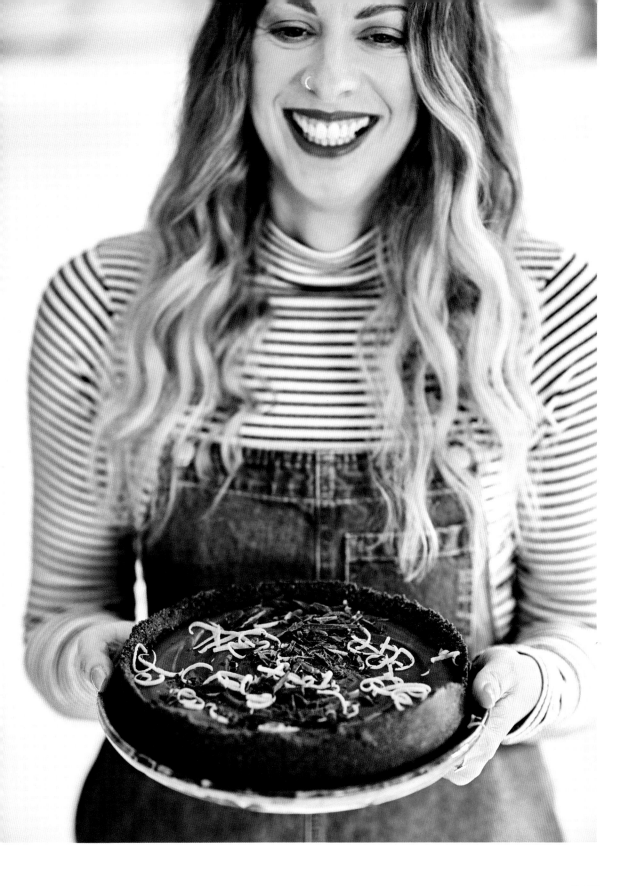

Arctic Roll

300g raspberry ripple ice-cream or dairy-free alternative
4 large eggs, separated
110g caster sugar, plus extra for rolling

90g gluten-free plain flour
1 tsp baking powder
¼ tsp xanthan gum
4 tbsp seedless raspberry jam

Prep: **15 minutes**
(+ 2 hours freezing)

Cook: **15 minutes**

Arctic roll is one of those school dinner staples I can remember from my pre-coeliac days. I've never seen a gluten-free version in the shops, but this summertime dessert is actually really easy and fun to make at home. In true retro fashion, I've gone for a raspberry ripple centre, but you can try it with any flavour you like.

Serves 12

1 Bring the ice-cream out of the freezer and allow it to soften until it's easy to scoop.

2 Place a sheet of clingfilm on your work surface and spoon the ice-cream lengthways along the middle to form a sausage shape about 25cm long. Roll the clingfilm around it and twist the ends together to form a smooth cylinder. Freeze for at least 1 hour.

3 Preheat the oven to 180°C/Fan 160°C/Gas Mark 5. Line a 38 x 24cm Swiss roll tin with baking paper.

4 Separate the eggs, placing the whites in a large metal, glass or ceramic bowl. Whisk with an electric mixer until they start to form stiff peaks. This is the point where you should be able to hold the bowl upside-down over your head and the whites don't fall out.

5 Gradually add the caster sugar to the whites while continuing to whisk, until they form glossy peaks. They're ready when you can rub a tiny bit of the mix between your fingers and it doesn't feel grainy.

6 Beat the egg yolks together in a small bowl, then pour them into the whites. Use a spatula to fold them in gently, being careful not to beat the air out of the mixture.

7 Place the flour, baking powder and xanthan gum in a separate bowl, mix together, then sift into the egg mixture. Fold in using your spatula again until there are no lumps of flour.

8 Gently pour the mixture into the prepared Swiss roll tin and smooth out with a spatula. Bake in the centre of the oven for 10–12 minutes. You want the sponge to be springy and lightly golden – if you overbake it, it will be more likely to crack when rolled up. Place the tin on a wire rack to cool for a minute or so.

9 Meanwhile, spread a thin tea towel on your work surface and lightly sprinkle with some extra sugar.

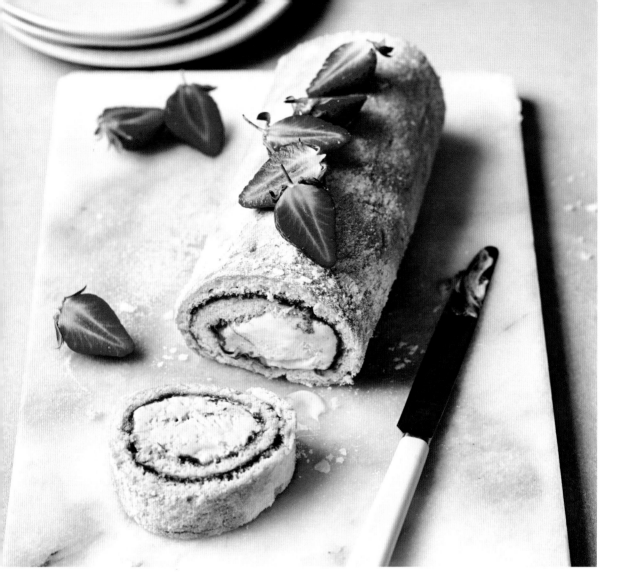

10 Gently invert the slightly cooled tin onto the sugared tea towel to release the cake. Peel off the baking paper, going slowly so you don't rip the sponge.

11 Using the tea towel to help you, roll up the sponge from the shortest end, then wrap lightly in the towel and leave to cool completely for about 1 hour.

12 Carefully unroll the cooled sponge and spread it with the raspberry jam. Unwrap the ice-cream, place it parallel to a short end of the sponge and roll up again. Wrap the filled sponge tightly in a sheet of baking paper, followed by a sheet of clingfilm. Place in the freezer for at least 1 hour.

13 Unwrap the roll and transfer to a serving plate, seam-side down. For bonus presentation points, trim the sides neatly and top with fresh strawberries.

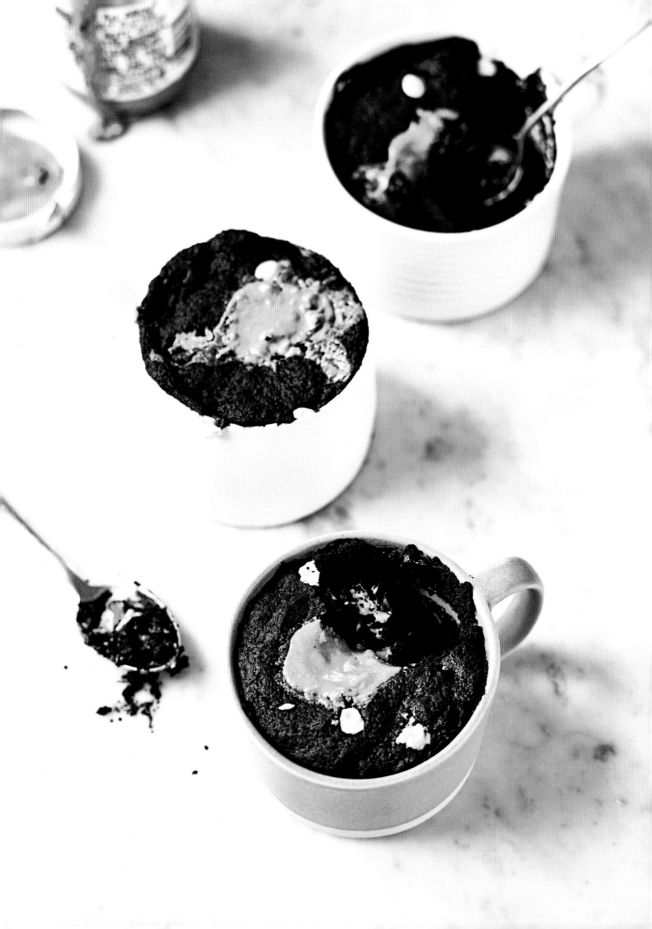

Chocolate Peanut Butter Mug Cake

30g gluten-free plain flour
20g cocoa powder
30g caster sugar
¼ tsp baking powder

20ml vegetable oil
3 tbsp cold water
1 tbsp white chocolate chips
1 tbsp peanut butter

Prep: **2 minutes**
Cook: **2 minutes**

You know those times when you really need something sweet but you don't want to bake an entire cake just to satisfy the craving? That, my friend, is where this single-serve, chocolate and peanut butter mug cake comes in. Gooey, delicious and thrown together in a matter of minutes, it's perfect for those nights when you want to indulge without any effort.

Serves 1

1 Place the flour, cocoa powder, sugar and baking powder in a microwaveable mug and mix together.

2 Add the oil and water and mix until smooth, being sure to get right into the edges of the mug.

3 Stir in the white chocolate chips, then plop the peanut butter in the middle of the batter and gently press down so that it is level with the surface.

4 Microwave on full power for 1 minute, then leave to stand for 1 minute before tucking in with a spoon. The cake should have risen but still have a lovely, gooey centre with the peanut butter mixed in.

TOP TIP

Try adding a square of chocolate or a dollop of chocolate spread instead of the peanut butter. If you switch the white chocolate chips for a dairy-free alternative, the recipe also becomes vegan.

Churros with Chilli Chocolate Sauce

250ml boiling water
50g unsalted butter
2 tbsp caster sugar
180g gluten-free plain flour
¼ tsp xanthan gum
1 large egg, beaten
½ tsp vanilla extract
1 litre vegetable oil, for frying

For the cinnamon sugar
100g granulated sugar
1 tsp ground cinnamon

For the chilli chocolate sauce
100g dark chocolate
Pinch of chilli flakes
100ml double cream

Prep: **20 minutes**
Cook: **20 minutes**

DFO

When you're gluten free, anything beige or deep-fried is often a treat – and nothing beats a stack of fresh, cinnamon-dusted churros. The simple, gluten-free choux pastry is piped straight into the hot oil, deep-fried and served alongside a chocolate dipping sauce with a chilli kick. It's the perfect dessert for sharing, and one you'll want to make over and over again.

Serves 4

1 Pour the boiling water into a non-stick saucepan over a low heat, then add the butter and caster sugar. Heat, stirring, until it comes back to the boil and the butter has melted. Set aside.

2 Mix the flour and xanthan gum together in a bowl, then add to the butter saucepan, beating with a wooden spoon until it forms a thick, dough-like consistency. Set aside to cool for 2–3 minutes.

3 Add the egg and vanilla extract to the pan, and beat using the wooden spoon until you have a smooth dough. Fit a large star nozzle to a piping bag and spoon the dough into it. Set to one side. Spoon the granulated sugar and cinnamon onto a plate and mix well.

4 To make the sauce, place the chocolate and chilli flakes in a heatproof bowl. Pour the cream into a clean pan and place over a low heat until hot but not boiling. Pour the cream over the chocolate and stir until it's all melted, forming a smooth sauce. Set to one side at room temperature.

5 Pour a 5cm depth of the oil into a large saucepan and heat until it reaches 180°C, or bubbles form around the handle of a wooden spoon dipped in the oil. Once hot, pipe 3 or 4 lines of the batter, about 13–15cm long, into the pan. Snip the ends with scissors to separate them from the piping nozzle.

6 Fry for 2–3 minutes, flipping halfway through, until golden brown on each side. Transfer the cooked churros to a plate lined with kitchen paper to absorb any excess oil, then roll them in the cinnamon sugar to coat. Serve the churros hot with the chilli chocolate sauce for dipping.

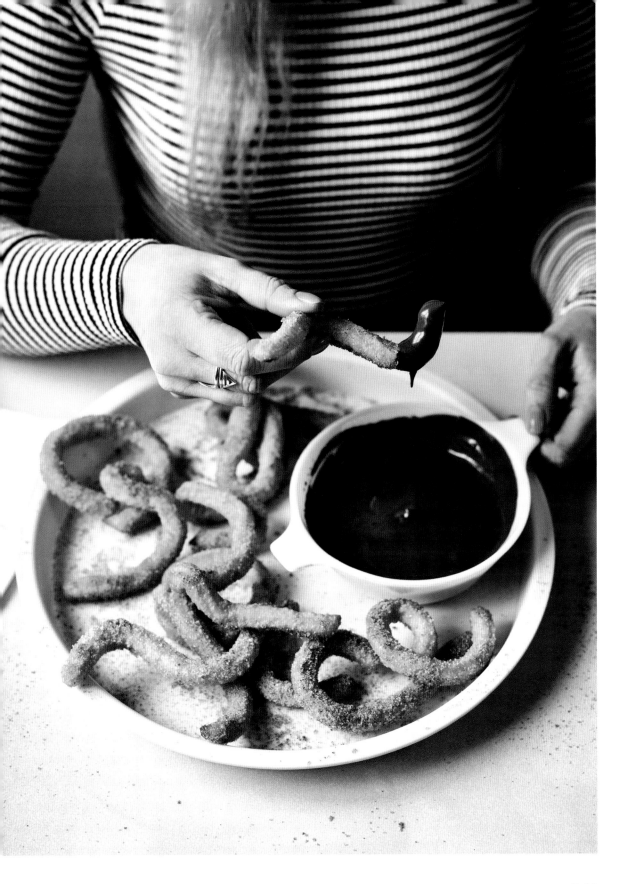

Index

Note: page numbers in **bold** refer to photographs.

Extra resources

If you enjoyed this book, you can find a whole wealth of gluten-free advice, tips and more recipes at **theglutenfreeblogger.com** or **instagram.com/gfblogge**r.

For more information on coeliac disease and living gluten free, I recommend the following places as trusted sources of advice:

- **Coeliac UK** (coeliac.org.uk)
  The UK's leading charity for coeliac disease. Their membership includes access to their Food and Drink Guide, which is updated yearly and includes a barcode scanner app. Very handy for shopping outside the free-from aisle and quickly finding which foods are gluten free and which aren't. They also have a freephone line staffed by dietitians, and a handy symptom checker for coeliac disease.

- **Guts UK** (gutscharity.org.uk)
  A UK charity that funds research into the digestive system from top to tail – the gut, liver and pancreas. It has information and fact sheets on all digestive disorders, including coeliac disease, IBS, IBD and Crohn's disease.

- **NHS**
  (nhs.uk/conditions/coeliac-disease)
  Provides an overview of coeliac disease, its symptoms and how the diagnostic process works.

About the author

Sarah Howells is a coeliac disease veteran of 20-plus years and runs one of the UK's longest established gluten-free food and recipe sites, *The Gluten Free Blogger*. She also shares gluten-free recipe videos on social media and YouTube under her handle @GFBlogger.

Diagnosed with coeliac disease in 2002, at the age of 12, she started *The Gluten Free Blogger* in 2009, while training as a journalist, as a way to connect with other people living a gluten-free life. Since then, she has built a thriving community of awesome, gluten-free superstars.

Sarah's mission is to ensure that being on a gluten-free diet doesn't mean missing out. As well as creating hundreds of tasty recipes, she advocates for better awareness and understanding of coeliac disease in the UK. She's also determined to show those struggling with coeliac disease that there is light at the end of the tunnel. Being gluten free is not a death sentence – it's the start of a brand new foodie adventure, and can be a whole lot of fun too.

Metric/imperial conversion chart

All equivalents are rounded, for practical convenience.

WEIGHT

25g	1 oz
50g	2 oz
100g	3½ oz
150g	5 oz
200g	7 oz
250g	9 oz
300g	10 oz
400g	14 oz
500g	1 lb 2 oz
1kg	2¼ lb

VOLUME (LIQUIDS)

5ml		1 tsp
15ml		1 tbsp
30ml	1 fl oz	⅛ cup
60ml	2 fl oz	¼ cup
75ml		⅓ cup
120ml	4 fl oz	½ cup
150ml	5 fl oz	⅔ cup
175ml		¾ cup
250ml	8 fl oz	1 cup
1 litre	1 quart	4 cups

VOLUME (DRY INGREDIENTS – AN APPROXIMATE GUIDE)

butter	1 cup (2 sticks) = 225g
rolled oats	1 cup = 100g
fine powders (e.g. flour)	1 cup = 125g
breadcrumbs (fresh)	1 cup = 50g
breadcrumbs (dried)	1 cup = 125g
nuts (e.g. almonds)	1 cup = 125g
seeds (e.g. chia)	1 cup = 160g
dried fruit (e.g. raisins)	1 cup = 150g
dried legumes (large, e.g. chickpeas)	1 cup = 170g
granular goods and small dried legumes (e.g. rice, quinoa, sugar, lentils)	1 cup = 200g
grated cheese	1 cup = 100g

OVEN TEMPERATURES

Celsius	Fahrenheit
140	275
150	300
160	325
180	350
190	375
200	400
220	425
230	450

LENGTH

1cm	½ inch
2.5cm	1 inch
20cm	8 inches
25cm	10 inches
30cm	12 inches

Acknowledgements

Until I started the process of writing a book, I never realised how many hands, eyes and amazing minds went into creating one, and I'm not sure the thanks I write on this page will ever do you all justice. But I will try!

First and foremost, to everyone who has ever visited my blog, liked a social media post, made one of my recipes or shared them with a friend – THANK YOU. Without you this book would never have existed. Not a day goes by when I don't think about how lucky I am that I can do this as a career and share my recipes with such a fantastic community. This book is for you and I think you are brilliant.

To my family – particularly Mum, Dad and Peter – thank you for being with me on my gluten-free journey from day one, for all the ingredient lists you checked and for always going above and beyond to make me feel like I was 'normal'. I feel very lucky to have always had such support from you all. Thanks too for willingly taking home samples of all the experimentations that led to the final recipe selection here – and for returning my Tupperware.

To Steve, my rock, thank you for believing in me, for picking me up when I didn't think I could ever finish this book, and for diligently eating both the recipe failures and successes. Your support kept me going and I couldn't have done it without you. Thank you, Janet, for letting me completely take over your kitchen – I promise I'll try to keep it a bit tidier now!

Clare, my wonderful agent and book fairy godmother, your initial belief in my idea gave me the courage to see this through, and you've been my biggest cheerleader throughout the whole process.

To my incredible Yellow Kite team – led by superstars Nicky and Liv – for believing in this book and in me. And for creating the most incredible dream team a girl could ask for.

From the very moment we 'met' on Zoom, I knew I wanted this book in your hands and you've both been super-supportive and made the process so enjoyable. Your guidance and wisdom have been amazing and I'm eternally grateful to you and everyone at Yellow Kite who has been involved in crafting, editing and publicising this book, especially Trish, Matt, Alainna, Emily, Vickie and Janet. You're all wonderful and I promise to bake you all (gluten-free) cakes to say thank you!

I cannot thank enough Steve for the beautiful photos, Esther for making my recipes look so gorgeous, Nikki for designing these stunning pages and bringing the whole vision together, Louie for your incredible eye for props, and Heather for making me feel so confident in the photos with your hair and make-up skills. You were the absolute photo shoot dream team. You made the creation of my first book the most joyful experience, and I feel incredibly lucky to have you all on side.

To my amazing friends who have supported me along the way, tried my sample recipes and been the best cheerleaders. Thank you all for being so understanding when I disappeared off the face of the planet for several months to write this and for always being so keen to try my creations and give feedback. You all rock.

Extra shout-out to Catherine and Kay for all your help testing many of my recipes on your unwitting families, and to Lauren for giving me your honest feedback every step of the way – along with the best salad dressing ever!

Finally, thank you to my wonky immune system for gifting me what many others might have called a curse. My coeliac disease is what brought my blog – and this book – to life, and for that I will be eternally grateful. I promise to continue giving my all to helping bring fun and flavour to everyone on a gluten-free diet.

First published in Great Britain in 2023 by Yellow Kite
An imprint of Hodder & Stoughton
An Hachette UK company

3

The authorised representative in the EEA is Hachette Ireland,
8 Castlecourt Center, Dublin 15, D15 XTP3, Ireland (email: info@hbgi.ie)

A CIP catalogue record for this title is available from the British Library

Hardback ISBN 978 1 399 72246 9
eBook ISBN 978 1 399 72247 6

Editorial Director: Nicky Ross
Project Editor: Liv Nightingall
Design: Studio Nic & Lou
Photography: Steve Joyce
Food Stylist: Esther Clark
Prop Stylist: Louie Waller
Senior Production Controller: Matt Everett

Colour origination by Alta London
Printed and bound in Italy by Printer Trento S.r.l

Hodder & Stoughton policy is to use papers that are natural, renewable and recyclable
products and made from wood grown in sustainable forests. The logging and manufacturing processes
are expected to conform to the environmental regulations of the country of origin.

Yellow Kite
Hodder & Stoughton Ltd
Carmelite House
50 Victoria Embankment
London
EC4Y 0DZ

www.yellowkitebooks.co.uk
www.hodder.co.uk